Notes on Paediatrics

Cardiorespiratory Disease

Alex Habel MBChB, FRCP, MRCPCH
Consultant Paediatrician, West Middlesex University Hospital;
Consultant Paediatrician, Great Ormond Street Children's Hospital,
London

Rod Scott MBChB, MRCP
Clinical Research Fellow, Institute of Child Health, London

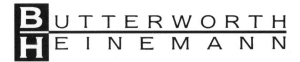

OXFORD   BOSTON   JOHANNESBURG   MELBOURNE   NEW DELHI   SINGAPORE

Butterworth-Heinemann
Linacre House, Jordan Hill, Oxford OX2 8DP
225 Wildwood Avenue, Woburn, MA 01801-2041
A division of Reed Educational and Professional Publishing Ltd

A member of the Reed Elsevier plc group

First published 1998

© Reed Educational and Professional Publishing Ltd 1998

British Library Cataloguing in Publication Data
A catalogue record for this book is available from the British Library

Library of Congress Cataloguing in Publication Data
A catalogue record for this book is available from The Library of Congress

ISBN 0 7506 2444 2

Composition by Scribe Design, Gillingham, Kent
Printed and bound in Great Britain by Biddles Ltd, Guildford and King's Lynn

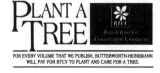

Cardiorespiratory Disease

Contents

Introduction to the series

Originally, *Synopsis of Paediatrics* was written with an overriding awareness of the need for a carefully focused textbook for practical work on the wards and in preparing for examinations using the problem-orientated approach. This series is a response to requests from students and postgraduates for easily affordable, updated versions of the most used sections. Thus the first section of each volume is an addition to the original text, containing embryology, recent developments in pathophysiology and disease management issues. Some sections in the Respiratory Disease volume have been completely rewritten.

As with the complete volume of *Synopsis of Paediatrics*, we have selected topics for their relevance to clinical practice. Doctors in training have told us that references are rarely consulted in textbooks, despite the preconceptions of reviewers (usually senior paediatricians), especially as up to the minute CD ROM searches have become so accessible. They are therefore kept to a minimum. The aim of the synoptic approach is to provide a digest on which the users can develop their clinical approach. A problem-orientated and systems method has been synthesized. In this introduction we will also touch on concepts that underpin this way of practising medicine in the last decade of the twentieth century.

HOW TO MAKE BEST USE OF THE TEXT AND IMPROVE YOUR SKILLS

Deductive reasoning in establishing a diagnosis

The success of a problem-orientated approach lies in sifting the information obtained from the history and signs to identify a problem or problems, then generating a list of possible diagnoses. The construction of a hypothesis of most likely causation is tested by deductive reasoning, answers to questions and findings of a positive nature tending to confirm, negative responses to exclude. Clinically 80–85% of diagnoses can be reached in this way, aided by clinical examination, confirmation coming from investigation where appropriate. Investigations should be selected to help confirm or reject the veracity of the hypotheses. When non-contributory or contradictory, review the history and findings and consider what further causes are possible. The alternative blunderbuss approach is slow, cumbersome and costly in time and resources.

Evidence based medicine (EBM)

'EBM is the conscientious, explicit and judicious use of best current evidence in making decisions about the care of individual patients'. Although this approach is traditionally held to be the scientific basis of our system of medical practice, a more critical appraisal of our use of examination, investigation and therapies has shown how shallow is that reality. We are increasingly asked to justify the clinical decisions we take, and this requires an awareness of published relevant clinical research experience. This is available on data bases such as the Cochrane Collaborative Project data base, and CD ROM and on-line computer searches of the journals. The aim is to integrate the best external evidence with individual clinical expertise. It also covers accuracy of diagnostic tests, prognosis, and physical therapies. We draw attention to this important development to orientate the student, be it at an undergraduate or postgraduate level, to the need to familiarize himself with this concept.

Reference

British Medical Journal (1996) Leader. Evidence based medicine: what it is and what it isn't. **312**, 71–72

Greenhalgh T (1997) How to read a paper. *The Basics of Evidence Based Medicine.* London: British Medical Journal

Acknowledgements

We wish to thank Dr George Sandor for reviewing the cardiology section and making valuable suggestions, the Editor of The British Medical Journal and Dr M Rosenthal for giving permission to reproduce figures.

Thanks also to Susan Devlin, our editor. Without her these slim volumes would not have been produced.

Abbreviations

Abbreviations have been kept to a minimum, and the following will be found in the text:

AD Autosomal dominant inheritance
AR Autosomal recessive inheritance
CT Computerized tomography
EEG Electroencephalograph
ESR Erythrocyte sedimentation rate
FBC Full blood count
LP Lumbar puncture
MRI Magnetic resonance imaging
US Ultrasound
WBC White blood count
XL Sex linked inheritance

Chapter 1

Respiratory disease

PHYSIOLOGY OF BREATHING

Respiratory physiology is the basis of lung function tests. Appreciation of the mechanism of respiration is fundamental to understanding.

In health, inspiration is an active process requiring energy expenditure, whereas expiration is a passive process when at rest.

Lung volumes

1   Total lung capacity: the volume of gas in the lungs and airways *after a full inspiration*.
2   Residual volume: the volume of gas left in the lungs *after forced expiration*.
3   Functional residual capacity: the volume of gas left in the lungs and airways *after normal expiration*.
4   Forced vital capacity (FVC): total lung capacity minus residual volume (FVC = 1 − 2).
5   Tidal volume: the average volume of a number of normal breaths.
6   Inspiratory capacity: the volume of gas that can be maximally inspired from normal expiration.
7   Inspiratory reserve volume: inspiratory capacity minus tidal volume (IRV = 6 − 5).
8   Expiratory reserve volume: the volume of gas that can be forcefully expired from the end of *normal* expiration.
9   Forced expiratory volume in one second (FEV_1): the volume of air that can forcefully be expelled in one second.

Obstructive lung disease, e.g. asthma, cystic fibrosis: FEV_1 decreases while FVC is normal.

Restrictive lung disease, e.g. fibrosing alveolitis: FEV_1 and FVC are both decreased.

EMBRYOLOGY

Development of the trachea

There is initial outpouching of the primitive foregut with subsequent separation from the gut with formation of the tracheo-oesophageal septum. The epiglottis forms at the origin of the outpouching.

- Tracheo-oesophageal fistulae (TOF) result from incomplete division of the laryngotracheal tube into gut and respiratory epithelia, and failure of the tracheo-oesophageal septum to form.

Development of the larynx

This derives from the endoderm of the laryngotracheal tube. Epithelium divides very rapidly causing occlusion of the canal. Recanalization occurs by the tenth week. During this process the vocal cords are formed.

- Failure of recanalization results in the formation of a laryngeal web.

Prenatal lung growth

First stage (0–5 weeks): outpouching of primitive foregut. Epithelium and mesenchyme interact to allow growth. Progressive branching to the level of segmental bronchi occurs.

Second stage (5–17 weeks): pseudoglandular period. Further branching of bronchial tree. Mesenchyme develops into cartilage, smooth muscle and connective tissue. All major elements of the lung except those involved in gas exchange are formed.

Third stage (16–25 weeks): canicular period. Increase in number of and size of terminal bronchioles. Lung becomes highly vascular. Respiratory bronchioles increase in number. Primitive alveoli start to form.

Fourth stage (24 weeks to birth): terminal sac period. Saccules resembling alveoli increase in number. Blood vessels develop close contact with the saccules. Epithelium differentiates into type I and type II cells.

Congenital malformations of the lung

- Agenesis of the lung results from failure of outpouching of the bronchial buds from the laryngotracheal tube.
- Lung hypoplasia due to pressure from oligohydramnios or diaphragmatic hernia preventing branching before the commencement of the second trimester.
- Lung cysts result from dilatation of the terminal bronchioles.

The major respiratory determinants of mortality in very low birthweight (VLBW) infants are the presence of adequate pulmonary vasculature and adequate surfactant.

Postnatal lung growth

Growth continues up to adolescence.

Trachea diameter trebles, a further eight generations of bronchioles develop, alveolar size increases by a factor of four and there is a tenfold increase in the number of alveoli in the adult lung compared to the newborn.

The alveoli mature by developing an increased surface area. This occurs as a result of septa forming on the walls of the saccules giving them a more adult shape.

EPIDEMIOLOGY

Acute respiratory infections

Acute respiratory infection (ARI): pneumonia, bronchiolitis and acute obstructive laryngitis (AOL).

Mortality worldwide

In 1990, 3.6 million deaths in the under 5s, pneumonia in 80–90%.
AOL, usually occurring as a respiratory complication of measles, in 475 000, and pertussis in 205 000.

Aetiology

Worldwide: pneumonias – *Streptococcus pneumoniae, Haemophilus influenzae*.
Comprise 50% of all illness in children under 5 years.
Comprise 30% of all illness in children between 5 and 12 years.

Developed world

The majority of respiratory infections involve the upper respiratory tract but approximately 5% will affect the larynx or lower; 90% of all infections are due to viruses.

Infants have up to six upper respiratory tract infections (URTI) per year especially if they have older siblings.

Children up to 6 years of age have up to nine infections per year.

Adults can have four to six infections per year.

Lower respiratory tract infections (LRTI) are commonest in infancy with approximately 25 infections per 100 children per year. This reduces steadily until the rate is five infections per 100 children per year in adolescence. The commonest LRTI in infancy is bronchiolitis.

The incidence and pattern of respiratory infections is affected by both host and environmental factors.

Host factors

- Age – most serious respiratory infections occur under the age of 3 years.
- Sex – boys have more LRTI up to the age of 6 years.
- Obesity – more infections in obese children.

- Congenital malformations.
- Immune deficiency.
- Prematurity – increased infections in the first 6–12 months of life.
- Breast feeding – appears to halve the risk of acquiring respiratory syncytial virus (RSV) bronchiolitis.

Environmental factors

- Quality of parental care – good care decreases incidence of RSV bronchiolitis.
- Parental smoking – the incidence of pneumonia is doubled in the first year if both parents smoke and increased by 50% if one parent smokes.
- Exposure to infection.
- Social class – the incidence is the same but severity is worse in poorer socioeconomic groups.

Children and smoking – cost in health in the UK

A Health of the Nation target for children's smoking was to reduce it from 8% in 1988 to <6% in 1994. Among 11–15 year olds 12% smoked in 1994. This continuing failure to halt, let alone reduce smoking prevalence, condemns 4–5 million UK children to become regular smokers. One million will die in middle age, losing 22 years' life expectancy. 1994 Government initiatives to curb smoking cost £10 million, the same year it received almost £9 thousand million in tax.

Recent therapeutic advice

Croup – management with inhaled steroid

Mild to moderate croup improves when given 2 mg nebulized budesonide, which can be repeated at 12 h, and results in early discharge and reduced re-admission when used in the emergency department. It may have a place in general practice, provided a reassessment occurs 2–4 h after administration. It is as efficacious as 4 mg nebulized adrenaline. No guidance for combining these therapies is yet available.

Further reading

Doull I (1995) Corticosteroids in the management of croup. Leader. *British Medical Journal*, **311**, 1244
Fitzgerald D, Mellis C, Johnson M *et al.* (1996) Nebulised budesonide is as effective as nebulised adrenaline in moderately severe croup. *Pediatrics*, **97**, 722–725

RESPIRATORY DISEASE

Disorders of the respiratory tract are the commonest illnesses in the under fives, among whom there are 57 000 acute admissions to hospital and 700 deaths annually in the UK.

Risk factors

1 The respiratory residua of neonatal intensive care, e.g. subglottic stenosis and bronchopulmonary dysplasia, have become increasingly prominent causes.
2 More likely and severe in the very young, exacerbated by poverty and parental cigarette smoking.

Pathophysiology of respiratory disease in the growing child

1 Immunity

Initial lack of specific antibodies in the infant and preschool children may result in a respiratory tract infection every 2–4 weeks in the winter months, often brought home from school by an elder sibling. Breast feeding gives some protection against respiratory tract infection in the first year of life.

The lymphatic system is very reactive: glands in the neck and hilar regions readily enlarge; tonsils and adenoids are at their largest at 6–8 years (previously peak age for their removal!).

2 Lung development, airway size and resistance, respiratory failure

i Airway development is complete at birth (16 generations), but the alveoli continue to divide, mainly in the first year, to complete 24 generations. The powers of recovery from damage to the lungs are therefore greatest during that period. However, the collateral channels (pores of Kohn, canals of Lambert) are not developed before 4 years old, preventing diffusion and contributing to hyperinflation, CO_2 retention and segmental collapse in obstructive airway problems.
ii Peripheral airway resistance in infancy and early childhood is relatively high under 5 years old, and the lungs have less elastic recoil, making the work of breathing greater.
iii Airway resistance in disease: as resistance to flow is related to the reciprocal of the fourth power of the radius, narrowing can rapidly become critical in the small airways of infants and small children by restricting air movement in or out. Mechanisms:

   a. Intraluminal obstruction by inflammation or structural narrowing. As the air flow speed increases past the obstruction a wheeze may occur.
   b. The trachea and extrapleural bronchi have C-shaped cartilages, allowing dynamic airway compression (DAC) of the posterior membranous segment from surrounding hyperinflated lung in bronchiolitis or asthma (Figure 1.1). The abnormally soft cartilage in tracheomalacia also allows DAC.
   c. Interestingly, the spiral smooth muscle in infants' airways extends further down the bronchioles than in older ages, yet they usually fail to respond to β-sympathomimetics.

iv Mechanical factors contributing to respiratory failure

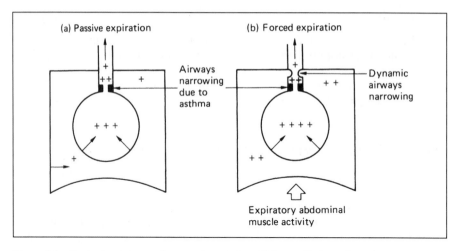

Figure 1.1   Expiration is normally a passive process. If the small to medium airways are partially obstructed the abdominal muscles are used to force the air out. A positive pressure gradient from alveoli to the mouth is established. At the point where the pressure is less than the surrounding pleural pressure the airways will be compressed. Now, the airflow across this point becomes fixed and the rate of exhalation is independent of effort

    a. The chest wall is more pliable in infancy, demonstrated by: Sternal recession: in upper airway narrowing (epiglottitis), and lung collapse (e.g. respiratory distress syndrome).
    b. The infant diaphragm has less type 1 slow twitch, high oxidative fibres and tires more easily than in older children and adults, who have more of these muscle fibres.
    c. Mucus plugging of small airways.

3   Investigations

X-rays

    i Chest. The thymus is large, jib-shaped or with a wave sign in infancy. It may 'disappear' radiologically in shock or cyanotic heart disease.
    ii Sinuses, age of appearance: mastoids 6 months, maxillary 1–2 years, sphenoid 3 years, frontal 5 years.
    Sites for the onset of sinusitis are therefore age related.
    iii Barium swallow for oesophageal reflux/tracheo-oesophageal fistula/ double aortic arch.

Blood gases, oxygen saturation

    i Ventilation-perfusion imbalance leads to hypoxaemia, defined as a $P_{a}O_2$ <7 kPa (50 mmHg). Pulse oximetry is often used to monitor oxygen saturation continuously, which should be maintained at 95%, equivalent to $Pa O_2$ 13 kPa (90 mmHg).
    ii Low carbon dioxide occurs in hyperventilation, mild asthma, or early salicylate poisoning.

iii Carbon dioxide elevation = respiratory failure (or rapid bicarbonate administration). In infants and children this equals a Pa_{CO_2} >6.0 kPa (45 mmHg), except in asthma when a 'normal' Pa_{CO_2} >5.4 kPa (40 mmHg) indicates respiratory failure as the Pa_{CO_2} is initially subnormal due to increased alveolar ventilation (and dead space).

Causes of respiratory failure must be due to obstruction, restriction, diffusion defect, or depression of the respiratory centre (Table 1.1).

Table 1.1 Causes of respiratory failure

Obstructive	*Restrictive*	*Diffusion defect*	*CNS depression*
Upper Epiglottitis, stenosis, aspiration, laryngospasm, Robin anomaly, choanal atresia *Lower* Pneumonia, aspiration, lobar emphysema	Pneumothorax Pulmonary oedema Hypoplastic lung Diaphragmatic hernia Ascites Small chest Muscle/nerve weakness	Interstitial pneumonitis Pulmonary oedema Interstitial fibrosis	Drugs Trauma Encephalitis Asphyxia

Respiratory function tests

See asthma p. 38.

Combined study: pneumogram = monitoring respiratory and heart rhythm and rate, blood oxygen tension/saturation. In near-miss cot deaths and cyanotic episodes it is used to determine the type of apnoea or bradypnoea, or abnormal cardiac rhythm. Add EEG or video surveillance in cases with neurology or when smothering abuse is suspected.

Others: sweat test, immunoglobulins, bacterial or viral antibodies, and precipitins for fungi, pH monitoring for acid reflux, drug levels, as indicated.

Examination

1 Appearance: pale, normal or cyanosed in air?
2 Listen for audible sounds

   i Stridor: mainly inspiratory if the narrowing is above the glottis. If below the glottis, expiratory wheeze or stridor may also be heard.
   ii Rattle: mainly an inspiratory sound, often easily transmitted and felt by a hand on the chest wall = secretions in the pharynx or trachea.
   iii Wheeze: occurs predominantly on expiration, synonymous with asthma but occurs in any partial airway obstruction.
   iv Snoring is due to upper airway pharyngeal obstruction. Sudden cessation of snoring despite visible inspiratory effort is a sign of complete obstruction and urgent need for a surgical opinion.

3 Cough. Preschool children swallow their sputum, and are often sick during coughing bouts due to the muscular effort compressing their stomachs. Abdominal pain from the muscular strain is common. A chronic, productive cough at that age should make one suspect cystic fibrosis/bronchiectasis.

4   Effort due to respiratory distress:

   i   Grunting on expiration against a partially closed glottis is seen mainly in infants with respiratory distress syndrome, and older children in pain, e.g. pneumonia with pleuritic involvement.
   ii Infants extend the neck to shorten airway; head bobbing suggests exhaustion. Children with upper airway obstruction lean back, head extended. In lower respiratory obstruction they tend to sit forward and fix the accessory muscles of respiration, leaning on their thighs or the furniture.
   iii Flaring of the alae nasi:

      a. Increased airway resistance: in obstructive airways.
      b. Effort: temperature, parenchymal infection, stiff lungs.

   iv Chest

      a. Intercostal recession: pulmonary disease, as collapse or obstructive airways.
      b. Subcostal recession: air trapping.

   v   Respiratory rate
       Upper limit of normal:
       Neonatal   50/min
       Infancy   40/min
       1–10 years   35/min
       >10 years   25/min

5   Finger clubbing:

   i   Pulmonary causes: cystic fibrosis, empyema, bronchiectasis, tumour.
   ii Non-pulmonary causes: cyanotic congenital heart disease, subacute bacterial endocarditis, inflammatory bowel disease, biliary cirrhosis.

6   Ears, nose and throat, and neck examination, are often left to the end of the examination, so we have dealt with them under upper respiratory problems.

7   Chest

   i   Shape: sternal recession develops in upper airway obstruction or widespread lung atelectasis in the very young with pliant costal cartilage. Barrel shaped/pigeon chest if hyperinflated.
   ii Movement: asymmetry may be visible, due to unilateral hyperinflation or collapse.
   iii Tracheal shift confirms (ii).
   iv Percussion: gently, as the chest wall is thin. Not of value in the recumbent infant, as the resonance elicited is from the mattress!
   v   Auscultation:

      a. Harsh bronchial breath sounds over the whole chest are normal in infancy, and in the midclavicular zone in early childhood.
      b. Coarse crackles (crepitations) close to the stethoscope are due to secretions in the bronchi, and often confused with referred sounds from the pharynx which are as if 'at a distance'. Both can also be felt by the palpating hands.

c. Fine crackles are fluid in the alveoli. Heard in pneumonia, with oedema fluid, and respiratory distress syndrome.
d. Wheeze: narrowing of the trachea and main bronchi, by inflammation or dynamic airway compression (see above).

UPPER RESPIRATORY TRACT

Improvements in health and health care have resulted in a decline in suppurative middle ear disease, and an increase in concern of the cause and effects of secretory otitis media on behaviour and speech development.

Examination of ears, nose and throat

1 *Ears*

i Shape: small, round, absent lobes in Down's syndrome.
ii Low set ears = below a horizontal line drawn from the outer angle of the eye, e.g. trisomies 13, 18, 21. In renal agenesis they may also be large and floppy.
iii Between the mouth and the tragus: congenital fistulae, papillomata due to first branchial arch (FBA) maldevelopments. Conductive or

Table 1.2 Relation of age to infectious respiratory illness

Age	Illness	Bacteria	Viruses
Neonatal	Pneumonia	E. coli ++++ Pseudomonas +++ Group B haemolytic streptococci +++	Respiratory syncytial virus (RSV) +++
Infancy	Pneumonia	Pneumococcus ++++ Staph. aureus +	Parainfluenza, influenza and RSV all ++++ Measles +++ Adenovirus ++
		Chlamydia trachomatis +	Coxsackie ++
	Bronchiolitis		RSV ++++
	Wheeze related viral infection		RSV ++++. Rhino-, parainfluenza, Adeno-, influenza viruses all ++
Preschool	Laryngotracheitis		Parainfluenza ++++ Influenza, RSV +++
	Epiglottitis	Haemophilus influenzae +++	Parainfluenza, Influenza Adeno-, RSV all ++++
	Asthma	Mycoplasma pneumoniae ++	Rhino-, RSV, Parainfluenza all ++++
	Pneumonia	Pneumococcus ++++ β-haemolytic strep. + Haemophilus influenzae +	RSV, Parainfluenza, influenza, all ++++
School age	Pneumonia	Pneumococcus ++++ Mycoplasma pneumoniae +++	RSV, Parainfluenza, influenza all +++
All ages	Otitis media, coryza, tonsilitis, pharyngitis	Pneumococcus ++++ Group A β-haem. strep +++ Haemophilus influenzae +++	RSV, adeno-, rhino- parainfluenza, influenza etc all ++++

sensorineural deafness is a recognized association of the FBA syndrome.
iv Mastoid for swelling and tenderness in otitis media.

Examination of the tympanic membrane (TM)

i   Demonstrate procedure to the small child on parent or doll.
ii Invite the child to hold the auriscope jointly with examiner, encouraging trust and a feeling of control.
iii Best view obtained: infant – pull ear lobe downwards.
                        child – pull pinna up and back.

Common findings

Grey drum, cone of light reflex = normal.
Dull grey + retracted (malleus is pulled in, and retracts posteriorly) = blocked eustachian tube.
Dull grey, bulging +/– bubbles or fluid level = secretory otitis media.
Pink around rim of TM   = crying.
Uniformly red   = acute otitis media.
Dark, almost black   = impending perforation or blood behind the TM.
Black hole   = perforation.
Bullae on TM (unusual) = *Mycoplasma pneumoniae*.

2   Nose

i   Shape examples: snub nose in the fetal alcohol syndrome, saddle in Down's syndrome, beak-like in craniofacial dysostosis e.g. Crouzon's disease: oxycephaly, exophthalmos, exotropia, optic atrophy, beak nose, prominent mandible.
ii Flaring of nostrils in fever, acidosis, asthma, pneumonia, acute abdomen, pain.
iii Discharge: whether purulent, blood stained and unilateral in foreign body obstruction or choanal atresia.
iv Internal inspection using an auriscope.

a. Look for nasal septum deviation (common), and at the mucosa which is often pale and swollen in allergic rhinitis.
b. Scars/ulcers in Little's area due to nose picking and bleeds.
c. Polyps associated with sinusitis, allergic rhinitis, and also cystic fibrosis. A sweat test is called for.

3   Mouth

See tonsillitis and pharyngitis for other abnormalities found on examination.

Causes of acute cough

1   Acute infections

    i Upper respiratory tract infection (URTI): coryza, tonsillitis, pharyngitis.

   ii Laryngitis, epiglottitis.

 iii Lower respiratory tract: bronchiolitis, bronchitis, pneumonia.

2   Asthma, wheezy baby syndrome.
3   Pertussis, and pertussis like, e.g. adenovirus, parainfluenza, chlamydia.
4   Foreign body.

Coryza

Usually viral, may be a prodrome to measles or pertussis.

Clinical

Sneezing, nasal discharge, sore throat.
Includes febrile 'cold' with systemic upset.
Duration 1–2 weeks. Sinusitis, otitis media common bacterial complications.

Management

1 *Infants.* Treat impaired feeding with 0.9% saline nose drops or topical decongestant 0.5% ephedrine/0.025% oxymetazoline nose drops, and painful distension of the TM with paracetamol elixir, for 2–5 days only; longer may lead to rebound vasodilatation (pseudoephedrine orally may cause hallucinations and is of little value).

2 *Older ages.* Paracetamol for fever, consider cough suppressants (e.g. codeine linctus paediatric has a place if it is keeping the child and family awake at night). Antibiotics are only indicated for complications. Antihistamines cause drowsiness, and have no objective benefit.

Tonsillitis

Usually viral (see Table 1.2).
   Swollen, red tonsils, often with exudate, fever, sore throat and cough.
   The only reliable sign is a red flush on the medial side of the anterior faucial pillars.
   Streptococcal infection is also characterized by high fever, vomiting, cervical lymphadenopathy and pinpoint haemorrhages on the soft palate and fauces.

Pharyngitis

Erythema of pharynx and tonsils, otherwise indistinguishable from tonsillitis.

Differential diagnosis

- Commonly influenza, adenovirus, the prodrome of measles (look for Koplik's spots).

- Glandular fever has a white membrane +/– purpuric spots at the junction of hard and soft palate, adenovirus a yellow exudate.
- Part of the presentation of scarlet fever or typhoid fever.
- Herpangina (coxsackie A) is uncommon: small vesicles surrounded by a red margin on the fauces; they burst and become tiny ulcers. It affects all ages, with high fever and lasts 3–6 days. Not to be confused with hand-foot-and-mouth syndrome (coxsackie A 16), which has vesicles on the tongue and buccal mucosae, backs of the hands, buttocks, and occasionally palms and soles.
- Diphtheria is rare, has a characteristic ulceration and grey web-like membrane which bleeds if its removal is attempted, foul smell, and 'bull neck' swelling of cervical glands.
- An easily removed tonsillar membrane is found in Vincent's angina. Do viral and bacterial culture of swabs and microscopic and bacterial examination of membrane tissue.
- Isolation of *N. gonorrhoeae* is highly suggestive of sexual abuse.
- Acute lymphatic leukaemia and agranulocytosis may present similarly, so a blood film, Paul Bunell or Monospot test is done in appropriate cases.
- Candidiasis in an older infant or child, +/– parotid swelling in HIV.

Management

Paracetamol, fluids. Penicillin for 10 days if streptococcal infection is clinically likely. Swabs for confirmation in uncomplicated tonsillitis or pharyngitis are not cost effective and cause delays.

A reduction in rheumatic fever may have resulted from the indiscriminate use of penicillin, but problems of allergy, diarrhoea and unrealistic expectations in the treatment of upper respiratory infection have ensued.

Diphtheria needs intubation, antitoxin (after testing first for sensitivity to horse serum), penicillin i.v., bed rest and serial ECGs for early recognition of potentially fatal myocarditis.

Otitis media

Prevalence

Two out of 3 children by 3 years, 1 in 3 of them having 3 or more. Peak at 6–36 months, declines after 6 years.

Factors

Poverty, day care/institutionalized, male, underlying abnormality, e.g. cleft palate.

Caused by URT viruses and bacteria; important bacteria are *Streptococcus pneumoniae* (30%), *Branhamella catarrhalis* and group A β-haemolytic Streptococcus (20% each), *Haemophilus influenzae*, *Staphylococcus aureus* (5% each).

Clinical

Severe ear pain during an URTI, with fever, hearing loss, and bright red bulging drum.

Infants may scream with pain, pull at the ear, and have constitutional upset. Myringitis bullosa is a bleb on the TM caused by *Mycoplasma pneumoniae*.

Spontaneous or therapeutic perforation with release of pus relieves pain. Mastoiditis is rare.

Management

i Antibiotic: penicillin orally, or parenterally for 1–2 days if very ill, for a total of 7–10 days. Ampicillin has theoretical advantages, not proven clinically, but is worth changing to if no improvement occurs after 1–2 days. Alternatives in penicillin allergy are erythromycin or co-trimoxazole.

ii Antipyretic/analgesic, e.g. paracetamol.

iii Decongestants, local and systemic, and antihistamines, are all of unproven value but often given.

iv Myringotomy for persistent pain and fever, and a bulging drum; rarely necessary, but allows the culture of pus and selection of the most appropriate antibiotic.

Recurrent acute otitis media including the use of grommets

Prevalence

About 30% of children have 3 or more recurrences. If pain is severe, or hearing loss >40 dB persists more than 3–4 months, grommets may be inserted; they are usually extruded after 6–12 months. Tympanosclerosis, with permanently impaired hearing, is a complication of repeated (usually >3) insertion or use of semi-permanent T-tubes.

Controversy

Although effective in the short term, with improved behaviour, concentration and education, there is little difference in these outcomes from the unoperated on prolonged follow-up.

Beware

Cholesteatoma is likely where an offensive smelling, thin, chronic discharge from a postero-superior or attic perforation (may be difficult to see) is detected. More common in cleft palate.

Secretory otitis media (SOM)

Prevalence

Affects up to 40% at 1 year, falling to 15% by 6 years.

Pathophysiology

Related to, but not necessarily caused by, infection, and eustachian tube malfunction (regularly in cleft palate, Down's syndrome). Negative middle ear pressure develops, and increased secretion from the lining cells of a fluid – thin, or thick and viscid, grey or amber. The TM has impaired mobility and hence conductive deafness is common.

Risk factors include mouth breathing, institutionalization, deprivation, and passive smoking.

Clinical

The TM may be bulging, showing bubbles of fluid behind the drum, or be retracted.

Behaviour disturbance (often due to deafness and subsequent frustration in communication), slow speech development, and intermittent deafness are each complained of and can be identified.

Investigation

1   Tympanometry is a test of mobility of the TM, using positive and negative air pressure transmitted via a snugly fitting ear piece. It requires no patient cooperation.
2   Free field testing using an audiometer, emitting pure tones, screens hearing.

The Rinné test (bone better than air conduction) is a simple if not wholly reliable screen for SOM producing >30 dB loss. Applicable in cooperative children over 5 years old.

Management

i   Decongestants, antihistamines and antibiotics are of uncertain value. However, nose blowing is important, as negative middle ear pressures are induced by sniffing.
ii Persistent symptomatic bilateral deafness: grommet insertion (adenoidectomy at the same time may reduce the number of reinsertions). Swimming with grommets *in situ* is now permitted by most surgeons, providing precautions (ear plugs and swim cap worn, no diving) are taken.
iii Check that hearing improves after (ii), otherwise a hearing aid for persistent conductive or previously unsuspected sensorineural loss may be required.

Indications for adenoidectomy and tonsillectomy

An appreciation that the tonsils are physiologically large in early childhood with a peak at 6–8 years has resulted in a reduction in unnecessary operations.

Opinion at present favours:

i Selective adenoidectomy with insertion of grommets for repeated otitis media or serous otitis media causing persistent deafness with impairment of development or education. Contraindicated in bifid uvula or submucous cleft, because of the danger of postoperative palatopharyngeal incompetence.

ii Tonsillectomy – absolute indications:

a. Obstructive sleep apnoea. Night time waking, coupled with day time somnolence. Parents note sudden cessation of snoring as the airway becomes obstructed by too large tonsils causing acute hypoxia. Commoner in Robin sequence and Down's syndrome and the over 18 months old.

Operationally defined as apnoeas of 10 s each, 30/h in 7 h of sleep.

Hypoxia and hypercapnia lead to pulmonary hypertension, and finally to cor pulmonale.

Adenotonsillectomy is urgently indicated.

b. After a quinsy (some argue this is only a relative indication).

iii Tonsillectomy, relative indications:

a. More than 3 *severe* episodes of tonsillitis per year for 2 years.
b. 5 episodes in 1 year with significant loss of schooling.
c. Recurrent otitis media.

Parents should be informed that the operation improves 60% of cases only. Those with simple repeated upper respiratory infections, allergies, etc should be dissuaded.

Further reading

Grundfast K M (1989) Recent advances in paediatric otolaryngology. *Pediatric Clinics of North America* **36**, number 6

Maw A R (1991) Developments in ear, nose and throat surgery. In *Recent Advances in Paediatrics 9*, (T J David ed) Edinburgh: Churchill Livingstone pp. 93–108

Chronic upper respiratory conditions

Causes of chronic cough

(Typical presentations and management discussed under individual conditions.)

1 Postnasal drip (some authorities doubt this is a clinical entity!): repeated coryza, allergic rhinitis, vasomotor rhinitis, sinusitis. Especially on being exposed to new pathogens by commencing school.
2 Asthma: may be the only symptom – after exercise, or at night.
3 Infection: viral (causing bronchitis in preschool and school ages), tuberculous glands (rare), *Mycoplasma pneumoniae*.
4 Unknown: a large group, possibly post viral.
5 Post-pertussis: usually early childhood.

6 Foreign body.
7 Recurrent aspiration syndromes of early infancy, with feeding and then vomiting.
8 Cystic fibrosis or lung collapse, rarely immotile cilia (Kartegener's syndrome).
9 Extrinsic compression of the trachea or bronchus by enlarged heart, glands, or tumour.
10 Smokers cough and psychogenic cough in adolescence.

Allergic rhinitis

Prevalence

10% of children.

Clinical

Sneeze, rhinitis, and itchy nose causing 'allergic salute' by rubbing the nose with the back of the hand, nasal voice, snoring, halitosis. Aggravated by smoking, or paint fumes.

Investigations

1 If suspected by history, skin prick testing may identify the cause.

   i   House dust mite, animal danders (perennial).
   ii Moulds (perennial + atmospheric changes).
   iii Pollens (seasonal: trees in spring, grasses in summer).

2 IgE and radioallergosorbent tests (RAST) are less specific, more expensive. Nasal provocation tests are rarely required.

Diagnosis

History confirmed by investigations, or exclusion of the allergen. Alternatively, empirically by the response to prophylaxis. *Vasomotor rhinitis* is a diagnosis of exclusion, when no allergen is found or prophylaxis proves ineffective. Systemic nasal decongestants (pseudoephedrine) may help and submucous diathermy works.

Management

1 Avoid the allergen, e.g. cat. Removal may be warranted, but the response is delayed as it takes at least 2 months finally to remove animal danders from the home.
2 Medication: duration as indicated by symptoms.

   i   Acute: decongestants for 5 days (longer may produce rebound hyperaemia).
   ii Acute or persistent: antihistamine, e.g. loratadine.
   iii Prophylaxis: local application of sodium cromoglycate 4–6 × daily or beclamethasone 2–3 × daily.

3   Anaphylaxis may follow hyposensitizing injections, which are therefore rarely warranted.

Chronic sinusitis

Definition

More than 3 weeks nasal obstruction and discharge, and postnasal drip manifest by laryngitis and cough night>day, often with a headache in older children.

Predisposing conditions

Allergy, cystic fibrosis, Down's syndrome, immotile cilia syndrome, immune disorders.
    Local factors: foreign body, deviated nasal septum, polyps, trauma, swimming, nasal decongestants, infected teeth.

Investigation

X-ray confirmation = sinus opacification, air-fluid level, mucosal thickening about 0.5 cm or more.

Management

1   Humidification, decongestants for 3–5 days only, amoxicillin or co-trimoxazole for 2–3 weeks, plus an antihistamine in allergic cases.
2   Antral puncture and wash out if no improvement in 5–6 weeks in maxillary sinusitis.

The neck

Presentation for assessment of a mass in the neck is common, pits or fistulae relatively uncommon. The precise anatomical site is a useful guide (Figures 1.2 and 1.3).

Cervical adenitis

1   Shotty cervical glands, with some fluctuation in size noted by parents, is common and normal.
2   Painful enlarging gland with fever occurs with suppurative lymphadenitis. Streptococcal infection is most likely. Consider Kawasaki disease.
3   Lymphadenopathy with intermittent fever in viral infections (infectious mononucleosis, adenovirus, cat scratch virus) and psittacosis.
4   Association with eczema, Still's disease, drugs, serum sickness.
5   Progressive enlargement suggests a tuberculous gland, or atypical mycobacter. If tuberculin test is positive and the gland fluctuant remove it surgically and treat.
6   Supraclavicular glands with progressive enlargement over 3 weeks

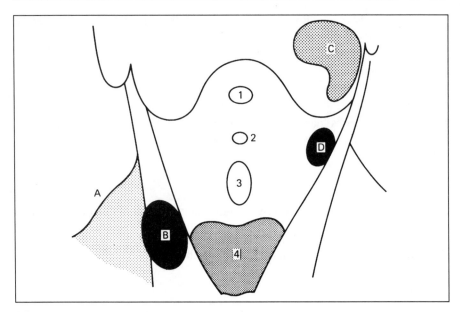

Figure 1.2   Anterior view:
Midline
1 = Submandibular lymph gland
2 = Dermoid cyst, attached to the skin, not the deeper structures like a thyroglossal cyst, number 3
3 = Thyroglossal cyst, moves upwards on tongue protrusion
4 = The thyroid gland moves upward on swallowing, distinguishing it from upper mediastinal glands that remain fixed
Lateral
A = Cystic hygroma
B = Sternomastoid tumour
C = Parotid gland
D = Jugulo–digastric gland

require Mantoux, ESR, FBC and biopsy for malignancy (typically leukaemia, lymphoma, occasionally metastases).

Further reading

Bain J, Carter P, Morton R (1985) *Colour Atlas of Mouth, Throat, and Ear Disorders in Children*. Lancaster: MTP Press (Simple, useful illustrations)
Isaacs D (1987) Why do children get colds? In *Progress in Child Health*, (J A Macfarlane, ed) **3**, pp. 38–46. Edinburgh:Churchill Livingstone.

Nose bleeds

Common in mid-childhood, usually from Little's area.
  History of bleeding, or of family members with bleeding tendencies, should be asked for.

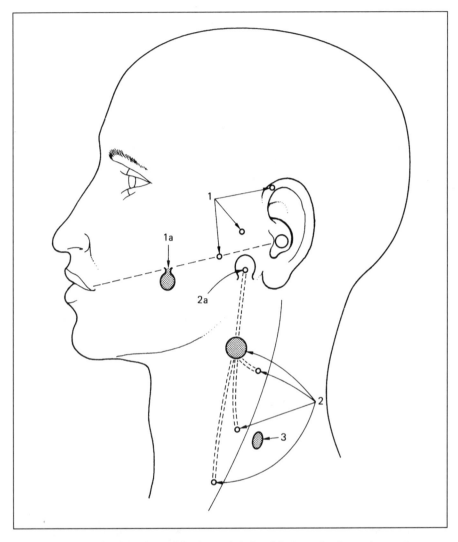

Figure 1.3 From the side, pits and fistulae and their origin from the first and second branchial arches and pharyngeal pouches
1 = First arch preauricular pits, and the area where they commonly occur together with 1a = first arch skin tag, along the line between the auricle and angle of the mouth
2 = Branchial cyst and external fistulous openings, anterior to the sternomastoid
2a = Fistulous internal opening through the tonsil
3 = Branchial remnant

Common causes:

1   Trauma, nose picking (bleeding is aggravated by low humidity).
2   Infection.
3   Allergic rhinitis: chronic nasal discharge, inflamed mucosa.
4   Foreign body: unilateral, purulent/serosanguinous discharge.

5   Bleeding disorders, vascular abnormality.
6   Tumours (rare).

Investigations

Visual inspection, FBC including platelets, and coagulation if appropriate.

Management

1   Applying 'clothes-peg' constriction of the anterior nares between thumb and first finger for 15 minutes is almost invariably effective unless an underlying clotting or vascular abnormality is present.
2   Continued/recurrent bleeding: chemical cautery, followed by electro-cautery if unsuccessful.

Stridor

Definition

   i   Obstruction to the larynx or upper trachea causing a predominantly inspiratory noise. Stridor predominantly on expiration is suggestive of subglottic narrowing.
   ii Croup is a 'brassy' cough +/– stridor due to acute infection.

Causes of acute stridor

1   Acute laryngotracheobronchitis.
2   Epiglottitis reduced in frequency since the introduction of Hib immunization.
3   Foreign body.
4   Measles, glandular fever.
5   Rare but important: diphtheria, retropharyngeal abscess, acute angioneurotic oedema, laryngeal burns.

Indications for intubation

1   Rising pulse and respirations, restlessness and cyanosis = hypoxia.
2   Progressive exhaustion manifest by quieter breath sounds, and shallower respirations.
   Generally blood gas analysis plays no part in management.

Airway assessment and management. Dos and don'ts

1   Epiglottitis

   i   Intubation for 1–2 days is the mainstay of treatment so admit to an intensive care unit immediately. To buy time, give nebulized adrenaline, 1 ml of 1 in 1000, diluted to 3 ml, effective for up to 30 minutes.
   ii If the child is well enough, X-rays may be obtained en route, but he must be accompanied at all times by resuscitation equipment and a competent physician.

Table 1.3 Features of epiglottitis, laryngotracheobronchitis (LTB) and foreign body above the carina

	Epiglottitis	*LTB*	*Foreign body*
Age	2–7 years	1–3 years	>6 months–4 years
History	Hours	1–2 days of coryza	Sudden onset, act of inhalation may be missed
Appearance	Pale, toxic, shock Sits, propped on hands behind, neck extended	Anxious/lethargic	Normal
Fever	+++(>38.5 C)	+	0
Voice	Hoarse, weak	Hoarse	May be aphonic
Cough	+	++	+++
Drooling, dysphagia	+++	0	0
Respirations	Laboured	Increased	Variable
Hypoxia	Frequent	Unusual	Variable
Epiglottis	Swollen, cherry red	Inflamed larynx, trachea	
X-ray of neck	Large epiglottis	Normal	May see opaque FB
X-ray of chest	Normal	Inflammatory changes in 50%	If FB moves below carina, then lung or lobe may overinflate or collapse
Blood culture	+ve	0	0
Intubated	60–80%	1%	?

iii Avoid excessive handling, leave putting up a drip and blood taking until the airway is secure, unless the child is not distressed or has collapsed already.

iv Acute laryngospasm and complete obstruction may follow pharyngeal stimulation so inspection of the oropharynx should only be done by experienced anaesthetic/paediatric staff as part of the intubation procedure. (An ENT surgeon should be on hand for emergency tracheostomy.) Proceed as follows:

a. Inhalation anaesthesia without the use of paralysing agents. The larynx may be so swollen that the only evidence of the airway is bubbles of air produced during the child's spontaneous breathing, which is abolished by paralysis.

b. Oropharyngeal tube is used initially, and changed for a nasoendo-tracheal tube after secretions have been sucked out and satisfactory ventilation secured.

c. Antibiotics: ampicillin resistant strains dictate the need for combining it (400 mg/kg/day) with chloramphenicol (100 mg/kg/day) or using a third generation cephalosporin (cefotaxime 100 mg/kg/day) alone, for 5 days.

d. Extubation 24–48 h later is usually possible. Depending on patient compliance, minimal sedation enables sitting up, and encourages spontaneous coughing to clear secretions.

2 *Laryngotracheobronchitis*

A progressive spread of the inflammatory process down the respiratory tree, due usually to viral infection. Only 1% of hospitalized cases require intubation.

Clinical

   i Coryza → laryngitis → croupy cough.
   ii Tracheitis: onset of inspiratory stridor after 1–2 days, worse at night.
   iii Bronchitis: respiratory effort increases as infection spreads down the bronchial tree.

Sternal indrawing seen, wheeze and coarse crackles heard.

Diagnostic confusion with epiglottitis occurs in the more severe, rapidly deteriorating cases, when the strictures regarding pharyngeal examination in epiglottitis must also apply.

Investigation

X-ray of the nasopharynx distinguishes it from epiglottitis.

Management

   i Mist. Although popular with parents, it is of unproven value.
   ii In hospital: minimal disturbance, parental presence for reassurance; oxygen for hypoxia via face mask or nasal prongs, if tolerated, with close clinical observation for further deterioration.
   iii Progressive hypoxia needs intubation as for epiglottitis. Adrenaline via a nebulizer has a temporary effect, but is useful while arranging intensive care.
   iv No antibiotics are necessary. Steroids advocated by some.

Duration of illness usually 2–3 days, occasionally 2–3 weeks.

Recurrent croup is characterized by a barking, metallic cough, and may follow LTB.

Characterized by mild URTI, followed by sudden onset of croup at night. The child is afebrile and anxious. Better by the next morning.

Often familial, asthma may follow.

3   Foreign body

Infants and toddlers eating hamburgers, ice lollies, small plastic toys, coins, pins etc; older children inhale peanuts, beans, seeds (Table 1.4).

Table 1.4   Characteristics of foreign body inhalation

Level of obstruction	Timing of onset	Symptoms
Laryngeal/tracheal		
i mechanical obstruction	Immediate	Cough
a. large, e.g. coin		Stridor, aphonia, dyspnoea,
b. oedema: small sharp object (e.g. egg shell, pin)		cyanosis
ii Chemical inflammation due to vegetable fibres, e.g. beans	Hours to days	Wheeze or pneumonia
Lower respiratory tract obstruction, inert material, e.g. smooth plastic or metal, roasted peanut, grass seed	Hours, days, weeks	Wheeze, unresolved infection or lung collapse, chronic cough and haemoptysis

Management

Any history of choking, cough +/– cyanosis requires laryngoscopy and bronchoscopy.

1 On chest X-ray the FB may be opaque.
2 X-rays on full inspiration and expiration may show a persistently hyper-inflated lobe if the FB acts as a ball valve obstruction.
3 These films may be impossible to obtain in small children, who should then be screened. Lung or lobar collapse with swinging of the mediastinum, or splinting of a diaphragm leaf due to ball valve obstruction, may then be seen when not previously visible on X-ray.

Management of other causes of acute stridor

Measles and glandular fever are unlikely to cause serious airway obstruction and can be managed conservatively.

Intubation to secure the airway must be considered in the following:

1 Anaphylaxis and angio-oedema (the latter usually shows as generalized swelling)

Due to allergen exposure in a sensitized child or family with C1-esterase inhibitor deficiency.

  i Clear airway. Lay child flat, legs elevated.
  ii Give oxygen.
  iii Drugs

    a. Administer subcutaneous (or deep intramuscular if shocked) adrenaline 10 µg/kg or 0.1–0.2 ml of 1/1000, and i.v. chlorpheniramine 5–10 mg.
    b. Repeat adrenaline in 15 minutes if no response. Steroids are not helpful in the acute situation, though i.v. hydrocortisone 100–200 mg is often given.

2 Laryngeal burns

Presumed present if soot is seen in the nostrils after a housefire.

3 Retropharyngeal abscess (rare)

Infants present with fever, drooling, neck hyperextension and a bulge of the posterior pharyngeal wall, pressing on the larynx. Danger of aspiration if it bursts, or erosion of the carotid artery. Incise under anaesthesia. Penicillin and flucloxacillin cover Group A β-haemolytic streptococcus and *Staphylococcus aureus*, the common pathogens.

4 Diphtheria (exceedingly rare)

See pharyngitis p. 11.

Further reading

Kilham H, Gillis J G, Benjamin B. (1987) Severe upper airway obstruction. *Pediatric Clinics of North America*, **34**, 1–14

Causes of chronic stridor

1   Airway narrowing above the larynx:

   i   Tonsillar hypertrophy.
   ii Tongue: Pierre Robin sequence, haemangioma.

2   Small or infantile larynx ('laryngomalacia').
3   Intraluminal narrowing at larynx and below:

   i   Subglottic or tracheal stenosis, haemangioma, cysts, laryngeal web, laryngeal cleft.
   ii Vocal cord paralysis: raised intracranial pressure, recurrent laryngeal nerve damage.
   iii Papillomata.

4   Compression of larynx or trachea:

   i   Vascular ring.
   ii Tumour, cystic hygroma, retrosternal goitre.

Investigation of chronic stridor

Indicated for persistent stridor or onset after 6 weeks old lasting >2 weeks. Not indicated for recurrent croup from URTI.

1   Barium swallow (see vascular ring), X-rays of neck for cysts, goitre, mediastinal masses.
2   Laryngoscopy with a light anaesthetic, or even none, to watch for vocal cord paralysis or the sucking into the airway of the folds of a small larynx.
3   Bronchoscopy if the lesion is likely to be below the cords, e.g. subglottic stenosis, haemangioma (like a cavernous haemangioma in the skin, it grows in the first 1–3 months, then slowly regresses by 2–5 years old).

Infantile larynx

Commonest cause of persistent inspiratory stridor in infancy.
Pathophysiology Disproportionately small larynx, its walls are sucked inwards more than usual, but there is no pathological softening of cartilage.
Clinical Appears aged 1–4 weeks, worse with URTI and crying, varies with posture. Micrognathia and Harrison's sulci are associated.
Investigation Confirm on direct laryngoscopy an omega shaped, anteriorly placed, small larynx, whose opening becomes slit-like on inspiration.
Prognosis Rarely obstructs, improved by 1 year, gone by 3 years.

Subglottic stenosis

Congenital, and acquired following prolonged intubation for respiratory support in extreme prematurity, just below the true cords.

Presents as croup if mild, or inspiratory and expiratory stridor if more severe. Laryngoscopy confirms. Avoid intubation, which may make matters worse; avoid surgery as widening occurs with growth.

Recurrent respiratory papillomatosis

Papilloma virus 6 and 11 infection found in the preschool age group. It may be acquired, at delivery, from maternal anal warts. Extends from the larynx downwards. Endoscopic removal, using CO_2 laser, repeated as often as necessary. Tracheostomy may be necessary. Lung parenchymal involvement rare, but may cause death.

Vascular ring

Due to embryonic remnants of the paired aortic arches encircling the oesophagus and trachea, and compressing the trachea between them. Tracheal stenosis is a common association.

Clinical

Persistent brassy cough and wheeze in early infancy.

Diagnose by a barium swallow to show indentation of the oesophagus by the aorta, and with a plain X-ray of the trachea, the aberrant vessel compressing the tracheal air column.

Acute cyanotic attacks/cot death 'near miss'

Finding a cyanosed infant or one in a pale, collapsed state, is not uncommon.

Exclusion of aspiration, acute infection (septicaemia, respiratory tract, meningitis), and consideration of intussusception, dehydration, or seizures, is mandatory. Metabolic problems, e.g. hypoglycaemia or inborn errors, may be evident from the initial investigations.

Repeated cyanotic or apnoeic episodes without obvious cause engender considerable parental (and medical) anxiety. Mechanisms proposed include:

1 Gastro-oesophageal reflux (also implicated in recurrent wheeze and stridor in infancy, but inconclusively). Not consistently demonstrated by oesophageal pH monitoring, but may be a cause in some cases.
2 Cardiac irregularity or vasovagal stimulation 'breath holding attacks' leading to hypotension and hypoxia.
3 Intrapulmonary shunting, associated with prolonged expiratory apnoea. Said to be provoked by emotion, pain, and cough, and also described as 'breath holding attacks'. No bradycardia or ECG abnormalities are found. A postulated precursor to sudden infant death syndrome, but controversy surrounds the original cases described (see reference).

Investigation

In addition to those on admission, continuous monitoring of heart rate and blood oxygen level for 24 h. In selected cases, barium swallow, oesophageal pH, or ECG and echocardiography.

Management

1   Monitoring at home with apnoea monitor or pulse oximeter or transcutaneous oxygen monitor. Parents should be instructed in basic resuscitation.
2   Antireflux posture and alginate or cisapride may be worthy of trial.

Further reading

Simpson H, Hampton F (1991) Gastro-oesophageal reflux and the lung. *Archives of Disease in Childhood*, **66**, 277–279
Stephenson J B P (1991) Blue breath holding is benign. *Archives of Disease in Childhood*, **66**, 255–257. Attacks the intrapulmonary shunt hypothesis, see associated articles

LOWER RESPIRATORY TRACT PROBLEMS

Radiological changes – causes to consider

A   *Recurrent or persistent lung field infiltrates and consolidation*

1   Infection: partially treated bacterial infection, TB, mycoplasma, psittacosis, pertussis, cytomegalovirus, Loffler's syndrome, *Pneumocystis carinii.*
2   Asthma.
3   Aspiration.
4   Foreign body.
5   Left to right cardiac shunt causing recurrent pneumonia.
6   Cystic fibrosis, bronchiectasis.
7   Malignancy: leukaemia (associated infection), lymphoma (recurrent infection and primary process), secondary deposit (nodular), Langerhan's cell histiocytosis (honeycomb).
8   Drug toxicity, e.g. nitrofurantoin, methotrexate.
9   Congenital: lobar sequestration (basal, in contact with the diaphragm), congenital lung cysts.
    Helpful pointers:
    • A history of previous similar episodes (asthma, cystic fibrosis).
    • Recurrent, persistent cough and breathing difficulties, perhaps despite antibiotic (infection, inhalation, congenital).
    • Vomiting/swallowing difficulties (aspiration), inhalation, ingestion of drugs, or findings of generalized/local suspicious lymphadenopathy or masses (malignancy).
    • A pansystolic murmur on auscultation.

B   *Asymmetry of lung field transradiancy*

Increased transradiancy

(A rotated chest X-ray makes interpretation difficult.)

1 Compensatory hyperinflation due to ipsilateral partial collapse or contralateral collapse in which case the contralateral lung is more opaque than usual.
2 Pneumothorax.
3 Lobar emphysema: foreign body, bronchial compression, congenital.
4 Lung cysts, pneumatoceles.
5 Bronchiolitis obliterans is included in MacLeod's syndrome of absent lung (post adenovirus or *M. pneumoniae* infection).

Opaque hemithorax

1 Pneumonia.
2 Aspiration.
3 Complete collapse of a lung.
4 Pleural effusion, empyema.
5 Haemothorax.
6 Diaphragmatic hernia, pulmonary agenesis.
7 Massive tumour.
8 Chylothorax:
      post traumatic/surgery.
      malignant obstruction.

Congenital abnormalities of the lung presenting as asymmetry in transradiancy

1 Lobar emphysema. Due to deficiency in bronchial wall cartilage, usually in an upper lobe, creates a ball valve obstruction, hyperinflation of the lobe and compression of the surrounding lung.

Presentation is usually neonatal with wheeze and respiratory distress, occasionally later, or may be asymptomatic.

2 Lung cysts – pulmonary, bronchogenic (lined with bronchial epithelium, usually mediastinal in position).

Presentation: (i) Compress surrounding lung tissue or bronchi, have rounded margins, may be fluid filled. (ii) Often become infected. (iii) Pneumothorax occasionally.

Lobar sequestration is intralobular, multicystic, not connected to the bronchial tree, and with systemic blood supply, in contact with the diaphragm, left>>right lower lobe; occasionally the lobe is outside lungs.

Presentation: cough, unresolved pneumonia, or incidental finding on chest X-ray. A CT demonstrates the consolidation +/– cavitation, and abnormal blood supply.

3 Diaphragmatic hernia usually presents in the newborn period, and is due to a failure of closure of (usually) the left pleuroperitoneal canal (90% cases) in the 10th week of embryonic life. The intestines in the chest prevent normal lung growth.

Treatment: surgery indicated for most cysts, even if not causing symptoms as they may well develop subsequently. Exclude staphylococcal infection, and hydatid disease in older children.

Pneumothorax

1   Trauma to chest wall or oesophagus, and surgery.
2   Assisted positive pressure ventilation.
3   Asthma.
4   Pneumonia with empyema, especially staphylococcal.
5   Cystic fibrosis (usually in adolescence).
6   Marfan's syndrome, Ehlers-Danlos syndrome.
7   Adolescent idiopathic pneumothorax.
8   Congenital lung cysts (see above).

Clinical presentation and management   Often sudden deterioration, unsuspected to be due to pneumothorax. Pain, breathless, cyanosis. Chest X-ray is definitive.

1   A small pneumothorax (<5%) may be left to reabsorb spontaneously, aided by breathing 100% oxygen.
2   Otherwise insert an intercostal drain connected to an underwater seal and apply continuous negative pressure (CNP) at 10 cm H_2O. 1–3 days of CNP are usually required for it to seal off.
3   Treat the underlying condition, give adequate analgesia, avoid respiratory depression.

Mediastinal masses (Figure 1.4)

Anterior

1   Lymph nodes:
    TB, leukaemia
    lymphoma.
2   Thymus: normal, tumour.
3   Goitre.
4   Dermoid.
5   Cystic hygroma.

Middle

6   Lymph nodes:
7   Bronchogenic cyst.
8   Post stenotic dilation of pulmonary artery (anterior) and aorta (posterior).
9   Pericardial fluid.

Posterior

10 Achalasia.
11 Duplication.
12 Anterior meningocele.
13 Paraspinal tumour:
    neuroblastoma
    ganglioneuroma.
14 Hiatus hernia.

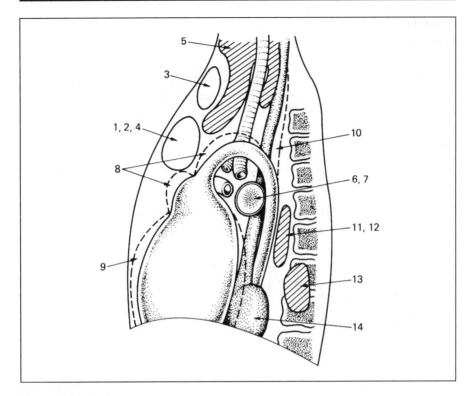

Figure 1.4 Mediastinal masses

Investigations are aimed at the particular part of the mediastinum. They include Tuberculin test, blood count and bone marrow, CT for cysts and tumours, spinal X-rays or MRI for enlarged intervertebral foramina or TB of a vertebral body; barium swallow for oesophageal disorders; thyroid scan for goitre; US for pericardial cyst; urinary catecholamines for neural crest tumours. Bronchoscopy, and thoracotomy may follow.

Wheeze in the first year

Important causes:

1   Acute bronchiolitis.
2   Wheezy baby syndrome.
3   Aspiration syndromes.
4   Bronchopulmonary dysplasia.
    Less commonly:

> Foreign body (above).
> Cystic fibrosis.
> Congenital airway or lung abnormality.

Acute bronchiolitis

Definition

Coryza for a day is followed by persistent cough, breathlessness, hyperinflation of the chest, and expiratory wheeze in a 1 to 6 (up to 12) month old. Fine crackles and cyanosis correlate with severe disease. Respiratory syncytial virus (RSV) is the usual cause, occasionally parainfluenza.

Epidemiology

1   1–2% of all infants are admitted to hospital with bronchiolitis. Occurs in winter to early spring.
2   Breast feeding and parental avoidance of smoking, each is protective.
3   Underlying congenital abnormality increases morbidity and mortality (see management (3) below).

Pathology

1   Inflammation of the bronchioles: secretion of mucus, necrosis of ciliated epithelium, and oedema of the submucosa causing airway obstruction.
2   Hyperinflation and patchy segmental collapse of the lung result, not helped by poorly developed collateral ventilation.

Clinical

1   As in the definition. Severe disease manifest as increasingly rapid respirations and cyanosis in air, inability to feed, head bobbing and unresponsiveness. 1% progress to respiratory failure.
2   Apnoea occasionally, especially in prematures.
3   Cardiac failure is unusual (but often considered due to liver depression secondary to lung hyperinflation), and secondary to underlying cardiac disease.

Investigations

1   RSV identified by immunofluorescence of nasopharyngeal secretions using specific viral antisera.
2   Chest X-ray shows square chest, horizontal ribs, hilar streaking, with subsegmental collapse or consolidation in 35%.
3   Blood gases usually show hypoxia. Hypercapnia common, the level occasionally higher than expected clinically.

Differential diagnosis

1   Wheeze related viral infection (a subdivision of which is the wheezy baby syndrome typically in a plump, less distressed, older at 6–12 months baby, chest X-ray less hyperinflated).
2   Asthma is unusual under 12 months, fine crackles are less prominent. The response to bronchodilators is haphazard.
3   Bronchopneumonia may also be caused by RSV, but the infant is more

ill, fever >38°C, no wheeze, fine crackles more localized; chest X-ray differentiates.
4 Cystic fibrosis is similar, but may wheeze for prolonged period.
5 Heart failure: has a very rapid pulse, and liver enlargement which can be differentiated from the downward displacement in bronchiolitis by chest X-ray or ultrasound.

Management

1 Admit to hospital if respiratory or feeding difficulties: minimal handling, suction of secretions if copious, feeding i.v. or via nasogastric tube if indicated.
2 Oxygen for pallor or cyanosis, via tent or head box. Assess severity with transcutaneous haemoglobin oxygen saturation (S_aO_2) by pulse oximetry.
3 Drugs: bronchodilators are of unproven benefit under 6 months, but ipratropium bromide inhalation, in the moderately severe, works in 20 minutes, and may help avoid mechanical ventilation. Ribavirin has some activity against RSV, needs a special nebulizer, and is very costly; reserved for the case with a complication, e.g. bronchopulmonary dysplasia, congenital heart disease, cystic fibrosis, immune deficiency. Antibiotics are not often indicated, nor digoxin or diuretics.
4 Mechanical ventilation. Note that elevated P_aCO_2 is common; blood gases are less important than signs of exhaustion, recurrent prolonged apnoea, or cerebral hypoxia, as indicators of need.

Prognosis

Death is rare, and associated with congenital malformations. Recovery occurs in 7–10 days, occasionally longer. Recurrence of wheeze in 50–75% (wheezy baby syndrome). Abnormal lung function tests may persist for years. A family history of atopy is not more likely, nor a tendency to asthma later.

Wheeze related viral infection (early asthma?)

Definition

Wheeze related viral infection (WRVI) is due to acute viral bronchiolitis, and more likely in the overweight baby, with no increased atopic history.
    Impossible to differentiate from asthma initially, but the latter is likely after repeated recurrences, or seen to be responsive to anti-asthma therapy, especially if eczema is present.

Controversy

WRVI is often a retrospective diagnosis, due to its subsiding by 1–2 years, whereas atopic asthma usually develops after this age.
    One view of wheezing children under 3 is that they are all asthmatic, the non-atopic representing a subgroup with age-limited increased bronchial responsiveness to a trigger such as viral infections, as in bronchiolitis and WRVI. Others, with an atopic background, also wheeze to the same triggers

but develop airway sensitization to aeroallergens, and become classic asthmatics later.

Management

Ipratropium bromide is effective in 40% of wheezy infants. Prophylactic budesonide via a spacer device with a closely fitting face mask reduces the frequency of recurrence, although there are fears of adrenal suppression and growth retardation.

Prognosis

Subsides by 1–3 years old.

Further reading

Leader (1989) Inhaled steroids and recurrent wheeze after bronchiolitis. *Lancet*, i, 999–1000
Milner A D (1989) Acute bronchiolitis in infancy: treatment and prognosis. *Thorax*, **44**, 1–5
Wilson N M (1989) Wheezy bronchitis revisited. *Archives of Disease in Childhood*, **64**, 1191–1199

Aspiration pneumonitis

Definition

Inhalation of milk, commonly, causing an acute inflammatory reaction within the bronchi.

Pathophysiology (and relative frequency)

1   Mouth: structural abnormality (uncommon) e.g. cleft palate.
2   Tongue and pharyngeal muscles: weakness or incoordination of sucking and swallowing (frequent), e.g. prematurity, cerebral palsy, CNS depression from drugs, epilepsy.
3   Gastro-oesophageal reflux (fairly frequent) from hiatus hernia or persistent vomiting, e.g. pertussis. Rarely due to a motility disorder like achalasia, or Sandifer's syndrome of torticollis and cerebral palsy.
4   Fistulae of oesophagus (rare), e.g. H-type fistula.

Clinical

Symptoms comprise vomiting or regurgitation, apnoea or cough during feeds, or acute cough and wheeze without URTI.

Recurrent aspiration may lead to interstitial pneumonia, secondary bacterial infection, and eventually even bronchiectasis.

Characteristically the baby is 'propped bottle fed' and has right upper lobe involvement on X-ray.

Diagnosis

1   Observe feeding. Evaluate neurology for cerebral palsy and motor weakness.

2   A chest X-ray typically shows inflammatory changes in the upper lobes.
3   Fat laden macrophages in tracheal aspirate likely.
4   Confirmation of reflux by pH studies or barium swallow.

Main differential is the presence of wheeze and fine crackles of asthma due to viral infections. (Reflux of acid into the oesophagus as a precipitant of asthma has not been convincingly demonstrated.) Recurrent cough has many causes.

Management

1   Antibiotics, physiotherapy.
2   Treat the underlying disorder by medication or surgery:

   i Antireflux: thickener (Gaviscon), motility agents (cisapride, domperidone). Stop drugs exacerbating reflux, e.g. theophylline.
   ii Surgery for medical failures (Nissen's fundoplication) and fistulae.

3   Support, e.g. for prematurity, cerebral palsy.

Further reading

Dinwiddie R (1990) Aspiration syndromes. In *The Diagnosis and Management of Paediatric Respiratory Disease*. Edinburgh: Churchill Livingstone pp 223–235

ASTHMA

Definition

1   Widespread airway narrowing which reverses spontaneously or with treatment, over short periods of time.
2   Clinical triad: cough, dyspnoea and wheeze.
3   Physiological triad: bronchiolar muscle spasm, mucosal oedema and increased mucus production.

Bronchial hyperresponsiveness can often be detected by challenge tests and reflects increased airway responsiveness to a number of environmental stimuli.

Prevalence and incidence

1   Atopy. About 30% of adults are atopic. In children, atopy includes infantile or flexural eczema, urticaria, hay fever, and asthma. About 70% of asthmatic children are atopic, and 70% of infants with raised IgE in cord blood develop atopic diseases later.
2   Asthma affects 10–15% of the population. Boys are more often affected than girls, but equilibration between the sexes occurs during adolescence.
3   The cumulative incidence of wheezing is 18% by age 7, 24% by age 16.

Increasing prevalence?

Over a 40-year period, a three-fold rise in the prevalence of asthma (or wheeze labelled as asthma) in preschool children has been reported. In childhood, 80% develop symptoms by 5 years old. Community studies confirm underdiagnosis occurs unless the appropriate questions are asked. Major factors possibly implicated in this rise include indoor aero-allergens, reduced exposure to infections and changes in diet. Only 4–6% of UK children receive regular medical supervision and is generally considered to indicate undertreatment.

Hospital admissions doubled in the 1980s, levelling off in the early 1990s. Failure to reduce the number of deaths from asthma in 1980–90 compares unfavourably with an overall fall of 24% for 'all causes' in the same decade.

Morbidity and mortality

1% of children with asthma are admitted to hospital annually.
Status asthmaticus causes 50 child deaths per year in the UK.

Aetiology

1   Constitutional (i.e. predisposition in that individual).
2   Atopy (inherited autosomal dominant with variable expression) = production of IgE antibody to common environmental allergens, especially those that are inhaled.

Both types have a tendency to bronchial hyperresponsiveness induced by precipitants. The commonest are respiratory infection and atopy or allergy.

Controversy

Genetic family studies implicate chromosome 5 (asthma and IgE), and chromosome 11 (atopy). Not all accept that the most significant gene locus for most asthmatics has been identified.

Pathophysiology of bronchoconstriction

Cellular level

Can be identified as acute and late phases, and chronic changes, each of which acts to produce or perpetuate wheeze.

1   Acute phase onset in minutes = bronchospasm
    Trigger stimulus

    i   of IgE antibody by antigen (type I reaction)
        → histamine and leukotrienes release (bronchoconstrictors from mast cells).
and/or
    ii increased airway receptor hyperresponsiveness (vagal reflex)
        → narrowing and shortening of airways.

2 Late phase, onset 4–6 h, lasting up to 10 days. Initiated by an allergen challenge, and thought to mimic the changes of chronic asthma (predominantly due to inflammation):

    i Mast cells and alveolar macrophages release leukotrienes, prostaglandins, thromboxanes → bronchoconstriction.

    ii Chemotactic factors attracting neutrophil, eosinophil, and macrophage migration, and platelet activating factor → inflammation and oedema of the airways.

    iii Chronic changes: damage to respiratory tract epithelium leads to increased bronchial hyperresponsiveness, maintained by the release of bronchoconstrictor substances, or by local axon reflexes through exposed nerve fibres, lasting for days or weeks.

Most have the acute phase (1) and recover within minutes, or a dual reaction of 1(i) and 1(ii), i.e. acute bronchospasm in an allergen challenge, with recovery within minutes, then a second episode 3–6 h later which is relatively resistant to β_2-agonists and probably causes 2(iii).

Nitric oxide (NO) in asthma

1 In hypoxia reduced production of NO may cause pulmonary vasoconstriction.

2 NO affects T-cell function, neutrophils and macrophages. It counteracts bronchoconstriction caused by degranulation of mast cells, and acts through non-adrenergic and non-cholinergic nerves as a neuronal modulator of bronchodilatation.

3 In higher concentration it is a vasodilator, causing plasma leakage, and a cytotoxin causing epithelial cells to shed. The rising incidence of asthma may be partly due to NO in car exhausts, cigarette smoke and gas cooker fumes.

Histological correlate

Chronic changes = inflammation

Increased smooth muscle bulk and number of submucosal glands produce mucus plugging of the airways, epithelial stripping and a thickened submucosa with cellular infiltrate and many eosinophils.

Clinical result

Wheeze is the result of intraluminal obstruction by oedema and mucus plugging, and, by muscular bronchoconstriction, dynamic airway compression of the intrathoracic extrapleural airways.

Precipitants of asthma attacks

1 Upper respiratory tract infections (80% of childhood asthma attacks) Mainly viral: rhino-, respiratory syncytial, parainfluenza.

2   Exercise (can be elicited in 80–89% of children)
Running exacerbates more than cycling, and in turn, cycling more than swimming. The response depends on inspired air humidity and temperature. Increase in receptor cells' intracellular osmolality triggers it.
3   Weather changes
Cold air, and humidity, increase fungal spores in the atmosphere.
4   Emotion
Laughing, crying, anger. Acute and chronic anxiety is important in some who subconsciously manipulate their families by illness. Established asthma may be worsened.
5   Aero-allergens

i   Seasonal: pollens, e.g. tree in spring, grass in summer, *Cladosporium* and *Alternaria* mould in autumn.
ii   Perennial: house dust mite, animals.

6   Food-induced
Cola drinks and ice, commonly, and cooking oil rarely, in Asians. Wheeze related to food intolerances are without other symptoms such as urticaria, and to be differentiated from those associated with anaphylaxis precipitated by shellfish or cow's milk protein.
7   Irritants
Painting, dust, smoking, paraffin heating.
8   Air pollution: minor effect only, on pre-existing asthma.

i   Particulate (London smog) size <10 μm, from burning fossil fuels, and diesel fumes (40% of particles in British air). Associated with increased mortality in asthma population studies in the USA.
ii   Photochemical (Los Angeles smog) from sunlight and car exhaust gases, nitrogen dioxide and ozone.
Some advise to commence or double prophylaxis and reduce activities such as sport until a few days after the episode of increased pollution.
iii   Gas cookers release oxides of nitrogen and may be particularly important in young children and their mothers.

Onset and course

Intermittent

1   Gradual onset. Cough for one day, progressing to wheeze within another, remitting by day 4, and better by the end of the week. In some recurrence is frequent, associated with respiratory infections, commoner in winter than summer and preschool age.
2   May be acute, even explosive, especially if sensitive to a particular allergen. Improves within 1–2 days.

Chronic

Milder symptoms are present much of the time, especially on exercise or at night. Particularly responsive to prophylactic therapy.

Symptoms

Age related. The natural history of atopic children shows a bimodal distribution, with one group who wheeze between 1 and 3 years old, and the other who develop wheeze after that age.

1   Infancy. Persistent/recurrent night cough, repeated wheeze with colds, persistent wheeze with obesity.
2   Toddler. Nocturnal cough is prominent, with recurrent wheeze on exercise, with emotion, and respiratory infection.
3   Children under 5 years old. Cough, may be the only symptom, often worse at night.

Associated symptoms

1   Breathlessness, episodic in nature. Expiratory wheeze. Abdominal pain and vomiting due to forceful coughing.
2   Repeated croup may be due to asthma.
3   Atopic eczema often improves during exacerbations, and vice versa, reason unknown.
4   Severe chronic asthma may stunt growth and delay puberty.

Severity

Mild = < one attack every month (75% of the total).
Moderate = > one attack every month (20%), no more than one a week.
   Both mild and moderate often have a marked seasonal variation.
Severe:

   i   Persistent symptoms, exercise limitation and abnormal lung function tests (5%).
   ii Uncommon: very infrequent severe attacks, even life threatening, but asymptomatic with normal respiratory function between episodes.

Impact of asthma on school and family life

Schooling

In physical education lessons 80% have exercise-induced symptoms, 50% are unable to complete. Up to a third of asthmatic primary and middle school age children miss more than 3 weeks a year and 12% lose 6 weeks. A third are woken more than once a week by their asthma. Sleepiness and inability to concentrate in class the following day is reported by 70%.
   This, with nocturnal wheeze in the early hours ('morning dip'), cyanosis or collapse are each indicative of the need for more effective treatment.
   Manipulative school avoidance is unlikely initially, but repeated illness with failure to keep up with class work may cause school failure.

Parental disruption

Employment: taking days off work at some time is reported by two-thirds of parents, though not regularly. A small number give up their jobs completely.

Social activities restriction is dependent on asthma severity, from not going out at all in a quarter for all parents, rising to a half if their child wakes every night due to asthma.

Further reading

Lenney W, Wells N E J, O'Neill B A. (1994) The burden of paediatric asthma. *European Respiratory Review*, **18**, 49–62

Signs

Mild to moderate attack

- Nasal flaring, prolonged noisy expiratory effort, raised respiratory rate, tracheal tug.
- Hyperinflated chest, plus, if chronic, sulci or grooves at insertions of the diaphragm produce a 'pigeon chest' deformity.
- Auscultation: widespread wheeze with coarse crackles, and often fine crackles in the preschool child.

Severe attack

- Cyanosis in air, grey appearance, progressing to confusion, or coma.
- Use of accessory muscles or difficulty in speaking in sentences are each equivalent to a peak flow <25% of predicted.
- Absent or quiet breath sounds in respiratory failure.
- Pulsus paradoxus >15 mm mercury (not a valuable sign).

Investigations

1   Forced expiration tests of lung function
    Effort dependent, highly reproducible in children over 7 years old, and sometimes younger. The normal values are related to height. Accept the best of three attempts. The most commonly used and useful tests in diagnosis and monitoring of asthma treatment are:

    i The peak expiratory flow rate (PEFR) is the maximal forced expiration, within the first one tenth of a second, through a Wright's peak flow meter or cheap plastic peak flow gauge.

       a. Normal values (Figure 1.5).
       b. PEFR below the 5% line *after trying*, requires action.
       c. The response to inhaled bronchodilators can be readily assessed. An increase of 20% or more is diagnostic, but failure to respond does not exclude asthma as bronchoconstriction may need more prolonged treatment.
       d. Variation in airflow obstruction is normal, with lower values of PEFR by 15% being found in the morning. However, low values (20% or more below the evening value) and 'early morning dipping' are important observations for management.

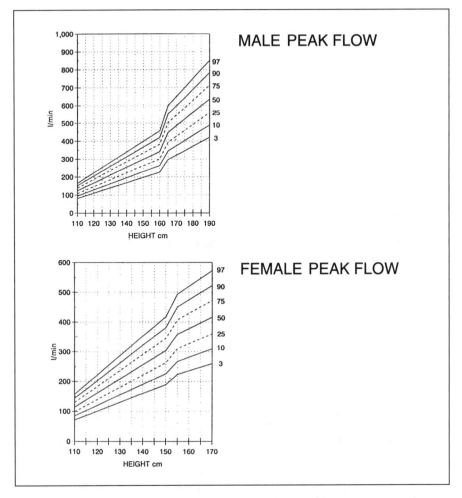

Figure 1.5 Normal values for white children in the UK. Note relationship to height and step increase related to the pubertal growth spurt. (Reproduced by kind permission of the Royal Brompton Hospital)

ii Forced vital capacity (FVC) is the total volume of gas exhaled during forced expiration. Reduced in small lungs, stiff lungs, scoliosis and neuromuscular disorders, e.g. dystrophies, myasthenia.

iii Forced expiratory volume $(FEV)_1$ is the volume of gas exhaled in the first second. (The $FEV_{0.5}$ is more reliable under 7 years old). Normally 80% of the FVC.

    a. Disproportionally reduced below 80% of FVC in airway obstruction, e.g. asthma, cystic fibrosis.

    b. An increase of 20% in FEV_1 after inhaled β_2-agonists confirms asthma. May fall to <50% of FVC during attacks, and remain low between them.

2   Bronchial challenge tests
These help to clarify or confirm asthma, identify trigger factors (inhalants, foods etc), and the response to treatments.

i   Exercise-induced bronchoconstriction.
   Method: exercise for 6–8 minutes on a bicycle or treadmill to accelerate the heart to more than 170 beats/minute. Then measure PEFR or FEV_1 taken at 0, 5, 10, 15, 20 and 25 minutes from the end of exercise (Figure 1.6).
   A positive response is a fall of 15% or more, usually found at 3–7 minutes.
   Cold air or nebulized distilled water ('fog') are also used in research as challenge tests.

ii   Histamine challenge for bronchial hyperreactivity, a research tool. Unfortunately, relatively unhelpful in defining the asthma 'grey case'.
   Method: using doubling concentrations delivered through a nebulizer for 2 minutes at 5-minute intervals until a fall in PEFR or FEV_1 of 20% occurs.
   The response in normal children is usually at far higher concentrations than those with asthma.

   a. This fall, the 'provocative concentration' or PC_{20}, in population studies, correlates with the minimum fall in PEFR for treatment to be required.
   b. Certain foods may increase the responsiveness in susceptible individuals (mainly Asians).

iii Inhaled allergens. Potentially dangerous, a research procedure.

3   Chest X-ray
Look for hyperinflation and segmental collapse.
   Not required in the routine assessment of the wheezy child, but only if symptoms are severe (pneumothorax or pneumonia present?), presence of prominent chest deformity, or a history suggestive of another condition such as cystic fibrosis, foreign body etc (see below).

4   Blood gases in severe asthma
Hypoxia occurs as PEFR or FVC falls.

i   pH falls: metabolic acidosis from hypoxia and work of breathing.
ii $Paco_2$ is usually low; if it rises to >5.4 kPa (40 mmHg), it is an indicator of respiratory failure which occurs in about 1% of hospitalized cases.
iii Pao_2 may fall significantly when β_2-agonist is given by nebulizer as airways open up in underperfused lung segments. In an acute attack Pao_2 may remain low for days due to ventilation/perfusion imbalance.

5   Other

i   Eosinophilia (>500 × 10^9/l) is commoner in atopics.
ii Positive skin-prick tests = test substance wheal >4 mm larger than control at 15 minutes, and suggests specific IgE is present. Late reactions at 3–6 h are also significant (see pathophysiology). Increase in size of reaction and range of allergens with age.

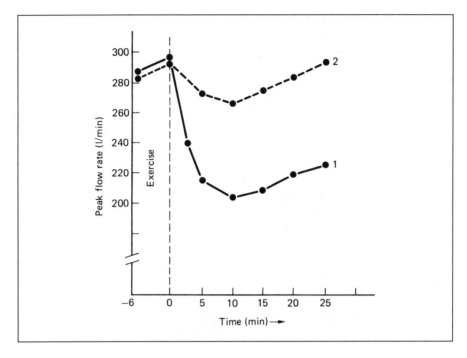

Figure 1.6 Exercise test
1. Positive test, fall of 80 l/min base line = 30%
2. Exercise repeated, with a negative test following pretest inhalation of a β_2-agonist

Skin tests (cheap) and blood radioallergosorbent (RAST) antibody tests (expensive) for house dust mite, pollens, animal danders and foods have a 50–80% concordance with symptoms. Positive results do at least support the history.

NB: 30% of the general population have positive reactions but only 25% of these develop asthma and many are free of any allergic symptoms.

Assessment

1   History

i   Age at onset, symptoms (may be persistent cough only), their frequency and severity.

ii   Other atopic features: eczema, allergic rhinitis, food allergies, irritability on allergen exposure. Allergens in the house (pets, plants) and bedroom (feather pillow or duvet, pet sleeps on the bed, dust collecting under the bed, in the carpet etc).

iii Seasonal variation and precipitating factors.

iv   Other causes of lung abnormality? e.g. neonatal intensive care, pneumonia, repeated aspiration, cystic fibrosis.

v Schooling attainment, time lost from asthma.
vi Exercise related wheeze, interference with sports and games.

2   Examination. In the assessment remember growth, pubertal rating, blood pressure (especially if taking oral steroids, when eyes should also be checked for cataracts).
3   Investigate appropriate to age and findings. Routine respiratory function tests require compliance!

Diagnosis

1   Repeated episodes of cough, dyspnoea and wheeze; +/– presence of infantile eczema and atopic family history.
2   A reduction of 15–20% in PEFR in an exercise test, or increase of >15% in PEFR following β_2-agonist inhalation.
3   Clinical response to a trial of a bronchodilating drug.

Differential diagnosis

1   Infants
   i Acute bronchiolitis: onset 1–5 days after the start of a 'cold', due to respiratory syncytial virus; fine crackles may be more marked than the expiratory wheeze.
   ii Wheezy baby syndrome/wheezy bronchitis: virally induced wheeze abates by 1–3 years.
2   Any age
   i Cystic fibrosis: failure to thrive, signs of bronchopneumonia, clubbing, abdominal distension etc.
   ii Foreign body. Always suspect this. If a likely object was handled and followed by an episode of paroxysmal coughing +/– cyanosis, investigate even if well on presentation.
   iii Recurrent aspiration: hiatal hernia etc, see Aspiration syndromes.
   iv Rare: bronchiectasis (+/– immotile cilia syndrome), airways compression from glands, cardiac enlargement, tumour, lobar emphysema, congenital weakness in bronchomalacia, post adenovirus infection in bronchiolitis obliterans, immune deficiency.

Management

General considerations

Guided self- or parent-management, as in many chronic conditions, is a partnership between the patient, the family, and the health professionals. The cornerstones are (i) understanding the condition; (ii) monitoring of symptoms, peak flow and drug usage; (iii) a prearranged action plan; and (iv) written guidelines.

1   Education. Assessment of severity and chest deformity. Frequent checks on inhaler techniques; theophylline levels to optimize treatment; check compliance. The aim is to facilitate a normal life.

2   Sporting performance impaired by exercise induced bronchoconstriction (EIB). Can be helped by pre-activity inhaled β_2-agonist or cromoglycate 5 minutes before. Lasts at least 2 h. Continuous prophylaxis with cromoglycate is equally effective. Nasal breathing reduces EIB. Short burst sports are best, though the child may 'run through' EIB, to a refractory state of reduced bronchial reactivity.

3   Environmental factors:

   i   Stop smoking. Avoid allergens, e.g. household pets (better still advise against their introduction into the house in an atopic family). House dust mite numbers may be reduced by impervious mattress covers. Humidifiers and ionizers are of unproven value.
   ii Hyposensitizing injections may allow a small reduction in medication, at the cost of a long series of injections and danger of anaphylaxis. Worth considering if a very significant reaction occurs to only one or two allergens, in the poorly controlled, severely affected child.

4   Emotional problems from within the family. They may respond to psychotherapy, which is not always available. An alternative option is 'parentectomy' by sending the child to boarding school in appropriate severe cases. Also monitor for bullying at school, and secondary gains from adopting the 'sick' role.

   Hypnotherapy and acupuncture are of unproven worth.

5   Home monitoring: the Daily Record Card. An important monitoring device, listing and grading the severity of symptoms (night cough, wheeze, sleep disruption, daytime cough, wheeze, exercise limitation), and their relation to twice daily PEFRs and treatment.

   Insistence on routine monitoring in the well child is unnecessary and psychologically undesirable.

Helping parents interpret the PEFR readings (Figure 1.7)

Predicted PEFR: use the mean value for height if no previous measurements are available when wheeze free (Figure 1.5). At other times, use the best achieved by that individual. The reason is that the normal range is wide, and the maximum for a slim chested, willowy Asian boy is very different from that for a solid Caucasian or Afro-Caribbean of the same height. Take the best of three puffs.

   i   PEFR below 80% of the predicted is abnormal. Start/intensify treatment.
   ii Below 60% significant airway obstruction. Intensify treatment, as agreed or consult with doctor.
   iii Below 25% is an emergency, requiring urgent medical advice.
       NB: The Wright minimeter overestimates by 3% (up to 10% in some hands), and should be borne in mind when interpreting results.

6   School: liaison with school nurse, ensure second inhaler is available, kept in the classroom or medical room, and that β_2-agonist can be taken before games/at breaks if necessary.

7   Outpatient review. Monitor the response to medication, its side effects, impairment of growth and school progress. The diary and a PEFR in the

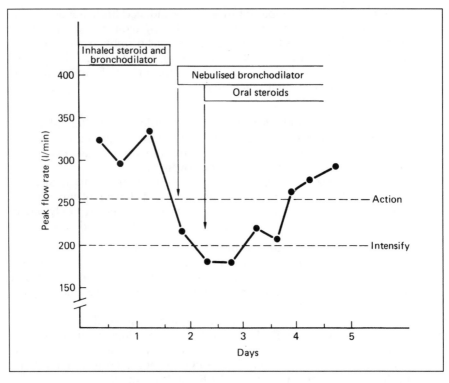

Figure 1.7   Marking a patient's peak flow chart to indicate when previously agreed action should be initiated. In this example, height was 140 cm, mean PEFR = 320 l/min
Action line (–20%) = 260 l/min
Intensification line (–40%) = 200 l/min
Danger (–75%) = 70 l/min

clinic gives an opportunity to see if the child's or parents' perceptions are exaggerated, accurate or dangerously inadequate.

Scores, peak flows, zones and management of asthma exacerbations

See Table 1.5.

Controversy: zones/scores or peak flows?

Considerable debate continues about which are the most suitable and dependable methods of monitoring and initiating treatment. The counter-arguments run:

1   Peak flow is effort dependent, and reflects performance technique. In addition the mini Wright meter readings are inaccurate by 5–10%. To initiate action at 80% and 50% of these PFs is pseudoscientific and potentially clinically misleading.

Table 1.5 Asthma treatment: interpretation of peak flows (PF) or symptom scores

Peak flow	Symptom score	Zone (National Asthma Campaign)	Action
80% plus	Under 6	1 green: seldom cough or wheeze	Continue usual treatment
<80%	6–9	2 amber: needs a reliever more than once a day	Increase inhaler preventer to twice usual dose for 1–2 weeks
		Cough or wheeze for last few days	Give reliever as needed
		Waking with cough or wheeze for last few nights	Contact the doctor in the next few days
<50%	9–12	3 red: needs reliever every 4 h	Give reliever as needed
		Coughing all the time	Continue inhaler preventer as above
		Too wheezy to run and play	Give steroid tablets as directed
		Waking each night with cough or wheeze	Contact the doctor
<30%	>12	4 purple: reliever lasts less than 3 h	Call for help from your: doctor/ambulance/go to nearest A & E
		Very distressed by wheeze or breathlessness	
		Too breathless to feed or talk	Give extra reliever, as often as needed, while waiting for help. Using a spacer will help. Continue inhaler preventer
		Lips go blue	Give steroid tablets are directed

Symptom scores on a scale of 0–3 for: night cough, night wheeze, daytime wheeze, daytime activity, nasal symptoms

2   Symptom based zones or scores are based on parent- or self-perception which can be misleading. If severity were underestimated this could (and does) result in inadequate treatment of life threatening attacks, prolonged reduction in activities, and increase in school absences. Judicious PFs in such a situation can highlight the child's true plight.

Findings from research

1   Guidelines for hospital admission:

PF can reduce unnecessary admissions: >60% of expected PF = unnecessary, 40–60% consider admission, <40% of expected PF = admission required.

2   Guided self-management:

Evaluation of a nurse led patient education programme when parents were given a self-management plan, compared with none, showed significant differences between the two groups in: less restriction of activities; fewer PFs <30%; fewer school absences; fewer home visits by GPs.

Further reading

Charlton I, Antoniou A G, Atkinson J, *et al.* (1994) Asthma at the interface: bridging the gap between general practice and a district general hospital. *Archives of Disease in Childhood*, **70**, 313–318

Table 1.6   Anti-asthma drugs, action, and important side effects (see status asthmaticus for i.v. drug guide)

Drug	Dose	Action	Side effects
β_2-agonist	e.g. Salbutamol: 200 µg 3–4/day inhaled, 0.6 mg/kg/day orally. Turbutaline 250–500 µg/dose 3–4/day inhaled. 75 µg/kg/dose orally, 3–4 daily.	Airway smooth muscle relaxes via cyclic AMP	Tremor, jumpy, tachycardia
	Salmeterol 50 µg twice daily	Not for immediate symptomatic relief	Commoner than with the other β_2-agonists
Cromoglycate	Inhaled: spincap 20 mg or metered dose 5 mg, either is given 3–4/day. May reduce to 2/day once symptoms controlled	1 Prevents mediator release from mast cells 2 Reduces reflex vagal stimulation	Nil
Corticosteroids	Inhaled* twice daily dose: i beclamethasone 100–200 µg/ ii budesonide 50–200 µg iii fluticasone 125–250 µg (half the dose of i and ii) Oral: prednisolone 1–2 mg/kg single dose or per day for 1–3 days	1 Anti-inflammatory 2 β_2-receptors more responsive 3 Phospholipase A_2 inhibited, reduces mediator release	Inhaled: oral thrush, hoarse voice, adrenal suppression? Oral: adrenal suppression and growth suppression if intake >0.5 mg/kg/day
Ipratropium	Maximum dose 40 mg Nebulized 100–500 µg. Metered 40 µg dose × 2, 2–3 per day	Atropine like, antivagal	Dries secretions
Theophylline	24 mg/kg/day in 2 doses Serum drug level maintained at 10–20 mg/l (55–110 µmol/l)	1 Airway smooth muscle relaxation by adenosine effect, not by inhibition of phosphodiesterase 2 Improves tired diaphragm contraction 3 Respiratory centre stimulant	GI: Nausea, vomiting CNS: headaches, bad behaviour school difficulties, seizures. Enuresis CVS: tachycardia arrhythmias

*Inhaled steroids: normal maximum dose is 400 µg/day for budesonide and beclamethasone, 250 µg fluticasone, but doubling or more of this dose is commonly required in steps 3 and 4 of management (see below)

Specific management issues

Nocturnal cough

About 5% of children with asthma present with cough; in the absence of wheeze categorization is difficult, and only 15% will show exercise induced bronchospasm and respond to bronchodilators. Troublesome persistent nocturnal cough in an atopic child or with a strong family history is an indication for a trial of β_2-agonist, oral (NB may prevent sleep) or inhaled, followed by inhaled cromoglycate or steroid, and finally oral theophylline.

Acute asthma management

Signs

- Too breathless: to talk, to feed
- Respiration >50 breaths per minute
- Pulse >150 beats per minute
- Using accessory muscles of respiration
- Classification by peak flow: PF <80% mild, PF <50% moderate, <30% severe
- Hospitalize if:
  unresponsive to β_2-agonist
  as bad within 1 h of its use
  previous severe attack requiring intensive support for collapse, or ventilation.

Life-threatening signs

- Cyanosis, silent chest
- Poor respiratory effort
- Agitation/reduced concentration
- Fatigue or exhaustion

Investigations

Blood gases are rarely indicated in initial decision making; X-ray chest if not improving after 30 minutes, or first episode assessed in hospital, or features of other conditions (remember other important causes of dyspnoea and wheeze in the preschool child, e.g. infection, cystic fibrosis, foreign body).

The acute mild to moderate attack managed in the community or primary care setting

β_2-agonist every 3–4 h:

- up to 10 puffs by MDI + spacer (+/– face mask) at 1 puff every 15–30 s or nebulized salbutamol 2.5–5 mg, terbutaline 5–10 mg (1/2 dose <1 year old).

  Improvement
  Continue 3–4 hourly, consider:
  Doubling dose of inhaled steroid
  Continued need 3–4 hourly after 12 hours?
  Start oral prednisolone for 1–3 days

  Failure to respond or relapse
  Increase frequency of reliever
  Start oral prednisolone
  Advise A & E attendance
  Call ambulance/go straight to A & E, continue β_2-agonist

- Antibiotics are rarely indicated yet often prescribed (about 80% of all attacks are virus associated, less than 5% bacterial).

Severe attack, failure to respond to initial treatment, transferred to hospital

- Oxygen, high flow via face mask.
- β_2-agonist via nebulizer driven by oxygen or equivalent dose via spacer device.
  Dose: salbutamol 2.5–5 mg, terbutaline 5–10 mg (1/2 dose <1 year old) or 10 puffs by MDI + spacer at 1 puff every 15–30 s.

- Prednisolone <1 year 1–2 mg/kg/day; 1–5 years 20 mg/day; older ages 40 mg/day.
- Monitor: pulse oximetry – admit if saturation <92% in air.

Life threatening features or poor bronchodilator response

- β_2-agonist via nebulizer driven by oxygen, every 30 minutes.
- Aminophylline 5 mg/kg i.v. over 20 minutes, then 1 mg/kg/h. Loading dose omitted if on oral theophylline. Alternatively, with poor response despite continuous nebulized β_2-agonist, start i.v. salbutamol 5 µg/kg over 5 minutes, followed by continuous infusion at 0.6–1 µg/kg/minute.
- Hydrocortisone 100 mg i.v. 6 hourly.
- Ipratropium 0.25 mg (0.125 mg in very young) added to nebulized β_2-agonist.

Continue to monitor oxygen saturation, maintaining it above 92%.

Note clinical features at regular intervals. Monitor hydration, as often dry.

Transfer to ITU accompanied by doctor prepared to intubate if:

- Worsening or persistent hypoxia or hypercapnia.
- Exhaustion, feeble respirations, confused or drowsy.
- Coma or respiratory arrest.

Discharge from hospital

Ensure:

- Stable on discharge medication for 6–8 h.
- Inhaler technique checked and recorded.
- Prednisolone course of 1–3 days provided or completed.
- Self-management plan or written instructions for parents.
- Follow-up arranged with GP or hospital.
- Direct readmission for any deterioration within 24 h.

Stepwise treatment of chronic (day-to-day) symptoms in children with asthma (British Thoracic Society guidelines)

Principles:

- Avoid provoking factors, e.g. passive smoking, do skin test for pets (especially cats) and house dust mite. If appropriate initiate action (remove pet, use bed covers, medical quality vacuum, remove carpets).
- Institute a guided self-management plan. Essential for steps 3 and 4 (see below), and those hospitalized for asthma.
- Most appropriate inhaler device for age and ability selected.
- Treatment started at the step most appropriate for severity.
- Prednisolone rescue can be given at any step, 1–2 mg/kg/day to a maximum of 20 mg/day under 5 years, 40 mg thereafter.

- Avoidance of provoking factors where possible
- Patient's involvement and education
- Selection of best inhaler device
- Treatment stepped up as necessary to achieve good control
- Treatment stepped down if control of asthma good

Notes

- **Patients should start treatment at the step most appropriate to the initial severity. A rescue course of prednisolone may be needed at any time and at any step. The aim is to achieve early control of the condition and then to reduce treatment.**
- **Until growth is complete any child requiring beclomethasone or budesonide >800 µg daily or fluticasone >500 µg daily should be referred to a paediatrician with an interst in asthma.**

Prescribe a peak flow meter and monitor response to treatment

Stepping down

Review treatment every 3–6 months. If control is achieved a stepwise reduction in treatment may be possible. In patients whose treatment was recently started at step 4 or 5 or included steroid tablets for gaining control of asthma this reduction may take place after a short interval. In other patients with chronic asthma a 3–6 months period of stability should be shown before slow stepwise reduction is undertaken.

Step 5

Addition of regular steroid tablets

Inhaled short-acting β-agonists 'as required' with inhaled beclomethasone or budesonide 800–2000 µg daily or fluticasone 400–1000 µg daily via a large volume spacer and one or more of the long acting bronchodilators

plus

regular prednisolone tablets in a single daily dose

Step 4

High dose inhaled steroids and regular bronchodilators

Inhaled short-acting β-agonists 'as required' with inhaled beclomethasone or budesonide 800–2000 µg daily or fluticasone 400–1000 µg daily via a large volume spacer

plus

a sequential therapeutic trial of one or more of

- inhaled long acting β-agonists
- sustained release theophylline
- inhaled ipratropium or oxitropium
- long acting β-agonist tablets
- high dose inhaled bronchodilators
- cromoglycate or nedocromil

Step 3

High dose inhaled steroids or low dose inhaled steroids plus long-acting inhaled β-agonist bronchodilator

Inhaled short-acting β-agonists 'as required'
plus either
beclomethasone or budesonide increased to 800–2000 µg daily or fluticasone 400–1000 µg daily via a large volume spacer

or

beclomethasone or budesonide 100–400 µg twice daily or fluticasone 50–200 µg twice daily plus salmeterol 50 µg twice daily. In a very small number of patients who experience side effects with high dose inhaled steroids, either the long-acting inhaled β-agonist option is used or a sustained release theophylline may be added to step 2 medication. Cromoglycate or nedocromil may also be tried.

Step 2

Regular inhaled anti-inflammatory agents

Inhaled short-acting β-agonists 'as required'
plus
beclomethasone or budesonide 100–400 µg twice daily or fluticasone 50–200 µg twice daily. Alternatively, use cromoglycate or nedocromil sodium, but if control is not achieved start inhaled steroids

Step 1

Occasional use of relief bronchodilators

Inhaled short-acting β-agonists 'as required' for symptom relief are acceptable. If they are needed more than once daily move to step 2. Before altering a treatment step ensure that the patient is having the treatment and has a good inhaler technique. Address any fears.

Outcome of steps 1–3: control of asthma

- Minimal (ideally no) chronic symptoms, including nocturnal symptoms
- Minimal (infrequent) exacerbations
- Minimal need for relieving bronchodilators
- No limitations on activities including exercise
- Circadian variation in peak expiratory flow (PEF) < 20%
- PEF ≥ 80% of predicted or best
- Minimal (or no) adverse effects from medicine

Outcome of steps 4–5: best possible results

- Least possible symptoms
- Least possible need for relieving bronchodilators
- Least possible limitation of activity
- Least possible variation in PEF
- Best PEF
- Least adverse effects from medicine

Figure 1.8 Stepwise treatment of children with asthma aged 5 years and over. Reproduced from the British Thoracic Society Guidelines with permission from the BMJ Publishing Group)

- Avoidance of provoking factors where possible
- Working towards a self-management plan
- Selection of best inhaler device

Starting out:
Patients should start treatment at the step most appropriate to the initial severity. A rescue course of prednisolone may be needed at any step (<1 year 1–2 mg/kg/day; 1–5 years 20 mg/day)

Step 1

Occasional use of relief bronchodilators

Short-acting β-agonists 'as required' for symptom relief but not more than once daily. Before altering a treatment step ensure that the patient is taking the treatment, the inhaler is appropriate, and inhaler technique is good. Address any concerns or fears. Mildest cases may respond to oral β-agonists.

Step 2

Regular inhaled anti-inflammatory agents

Inhaled short-acting β-agonists 'as required'
plus
(i) cromoglycate as powder (20 mg 3–4 times daily) or via metered dose inhaler and large volume spacer (10 mg thrice daily)
or
(ii) beclomethasone or budesonide up to 400 μg or fluticasone up to 200 μg daily. Consider a 5-day course of soluble prednisolone (dose given above) or temporary increase in inhaled steroids (double dose) to gain rapid control.

Step 3

Increased dose inhaled steroids

Inhaled short-acting β-agonists 'as required'
plus
beclomethasone or budesonide increased to 800 μg or fluticasone 500 μg daily via a large volume spacer. Consider short prednisolone course. Consider adding regular twice daily long-acting β-agonist or a slow release xanthine.

Step 4

High dose inhaled steroids and bronchodilators

Inhaled steroids (up to 2 mg/day) and other treatment as in step 3. Slow release xanthines or nebulized β-agonists.

Stepping down

Regularly review the need to decrease treatment and step down as indicated. Monitor all changes in treatment by clinical review.

Figure 1.9 Stepwise management of asthma in children under 5 years of age. Reproduced from the British Thoracic Society Guidelines with permission from the BMJ Publishing Group)

Notes on the management of asthma in children under 5 years of age

Step 1

Use inhaled drugs wherever possible. Bronchodilator syrups are much less effectvie than inhaled β-agonists and have more systemic side-effects.

Step 2

Cromoglycate is safe and helpful in many children and is still recommended as an optional first line preventive treatment. A therapeutic trial of 4–6 weeks is indicated. Start an inhaled steroid at a dosage appropriate to the child's age and size and the severity of the asthma. It may be necessary to start at a higher dose or to give a short course of prednisolone tablets for stabilization (dose given above).

After one month assess the effect on symptoms and adjust the dose. If control is not adequate, consider doubling the dose of inhaled steroids for one month. Alternatively, give a short course of prednisolone tablets, or consider introducing other treatments before increasing the inhaled steroid for longer periods.

Step 3

Inhaled long-acting β-agonists produce bronchodilatation in children for up to 12 h and inhibit exercise induced bronchoconstriction. More information about their long-term clinical effects is awaited. It seems likely that their role should be reserved for supplementing treatment in children already receiving regular preventer therapy.

Sustained release xanthines produce effective bronchodilatation but have appreciable side effects in up to one third of children (gastrointestinal disorders, sleep disturbance and psychological changes). They may be helpful, particularly for nocturnal symptoms, but monitoring of serum or salivary concentrations is recommended.

Step 4

Check inhaler technique, chart compliance.

Problems in the management of very young children (0–2 years)

- Recurrent wheeze and cough are associated with viral infections, often without a family history of asthma or atopy.
- Diagnosis relies almost entirely on symptoms, which may be very variable, rather than on objective lung function tests.
- There is a paucity of suitably designed and tested inhaler devices specific for this age group.
- Very few controlled trials of treatment have been carried out. Most treatments have poor efficacy, but should still be tried if indicated.
- The younger the child, the more other disorders may mimic asthma, such as gastro-oesophageal reflux, cystic fibrosis, inhaled foreign body, congenital abnormalities, and chronic lung disease of prematurity.
- Nebulized β-agonists in infancy may result in initial paradoxical bronchoconstriction and mild hypoxaemia. This does not seem to happen with a metered dose inhaler and large volume spacer and face mask, possibly because a lower dose is generally used. Anecdotal evidence suggests that ipratropium bromide may be more effective than salbutamol in the first year of life. There have been no controlled studies.
- Although doubts exist about the efficacy of ketotifen in older children, some benefits have been shown in infancy and it may be of some help in very young children intolerant of other drugs.

Before stepping up or down check

- Compliance.
- Inhaler device is appropriate.
- Technique is satisfactory.

A decision to step-up is based on:

- The presence of night-time or daytime symptoms. Persistent night cough or wheeze, and/or early morning cough or wheeze for two nights or more a week and not due to a simple cold.
- Wheeze or cough brought on by exercise.
- Need to use a reliever more than once a day or more than four times a week on a regular basis.
- If using a peak flow meter, reading less than 80% of the child's best 'blow', or the level set by the doctor or nurse, on most days.
- After a course of prednisolone consider: if the attacks last less than 2 weeks and happen less than 6 times a year is there a need to step up?

Step 1: Occasional use of bronchodilators ('relievers')

- Short-acting β_2-agonists as required, no more than once daily.

Step 2: Introduce regular inhaled prophylaxis ('preventers')

- Short-acting β_2-agonists as required, up to 4 hourly.
- Add *either* cromoglycate (powder 20 mg 3–4 times a day or inhaler 10 mg thrice daily) *or* steroid up to recommended daily maximum (400 µg budesonide and beclamethasone, 200 µg fluticasone.
- For rapid control consider 5 days of prednisolone or 2 weeks of double dose inhaled steroids.

Step 3: Increase dose of inhaled steroids

- Short-acting β_2-agonists as required, up to 4 hourly.
- Increase beclamethasone or budesonide to 800 µg or fluticasone 500 µg daily via a large volume spacer.
- Consider a short course of prednisolone.
- Consider regular long acting β_2-agonist or slow release xanthine.

Step 4: High dose inhaled steroids and bronchodilators

- Inhaled steroids (as budesonide up to 1000 µg 12 hourly) up to 2 mg/day.
- Regular slow release xanthines.
- Nebulized β_2-agonists.

Stepping down

Step down once control is achieved, i.e. if symptom free for several weeks or months. Decrease the dose of inhaled steroid by 25–50% steps every 1–3 months; once daily may be sufficient when on budesonide.

The drug delivery system

This is determined by age. Choosing an inappropriate method is a common cause of treatment failure and non-compliance.

Delivery systems for asthma treatment by age

1 Under 1 year: inhaled or oral?

β_2-agonists and ipratropium bromide best via a tight fitting face mask attached to a low resistance spacer (Aerochamber, System 22) or nebulizer. Under 18 months inhaled β_2-agonists may cause V/Q mismatch and so lower Pao_2; an oral suspension could be tried if treating a mild attack.

- Nebulized β_2-sympathomimetics should be driven by oxygen in critically ill infants. The rationale is that V/Q imbalance persists for 30 minutes after giving salbutamol, therefore it is unsafe to give nebulized salbutamol at home under 18 months of age.

2 1–3 years: inhaled therapy is superior

i Syrups have no real place.

ii Via nebulizer, driven by oxygen or air compressor (flow rate 8–10 l/minute) in a volume of 4 ml: face mask should be held as close to the face as possible, avoiding upsetting the child as much as possible. Any gap between the face and the mask reduces the dose inhaled very significantly.

Relief: salbutamol/terbutaline for the moderate/severe attack.

Prophylaxis: inhaled cromoglycate, nebulized budesonide.

In status asthmaticus: β_2-agonist, add ipratropium even though the effect is small.

iii Tight fitting face mask attached to a spacer (Aerochamber, Babyhaler, Nebuhaler) to deliver a β_2-agonist, budesonide, beclomethasone, or fluticasone

iv Coffee cup spacer in emergency – usually limited effect.

3 Preschool 3–5 years

i Metered dose aerosol inhalers (MDI) can be used by most children, via a spacer with mouthpiece, e.g. Nebuhaler/Volumatic 750 ml in size.

ii Others need a nebulizer (for β_2-agonist, cromoglycate, budesonide, ipratropium).

iii Slow release theophylline may have a place (see Treatment controversies).

4 Age 5–10 years

i Powder inhalation devices (β_2-agonists, steroids). A whistle attachment is a useful teaching aid. All require rapid active inspiration.

   a. PEFR of >60 l/minute is needed for the rotahaler, spinhaler, and diskhaler, inhaled over 3–4 breaths.

  b. PEFR of as little as 20 l/minute will activate the turbohaler.

  ii Breath-activated inhaler (BAI): minimal inspiratory effort needed is PEFR of 30 l/minute, with a long slow inspiration which should be held as long as possible (10 seconds is recommended). Suits 8 year olds and up.

  iii Spacers and nebulizers also have a place as ordinary metered dose aerosol inhaler (MDI) administration is often ineffective due to lack of motivation, or inability to coordinate.

5 Aged >10 years

BAIs and MDIs as well as the above.

Table 1.7 Table of devices by age

Device	*1–2*	Age (years) *3–5*	*5+*
MDI + spacer and face mask	1st	2nd	
MDI + spacer with mouthpiece	Poor	1st	If beco/budes >800 μg day or fluticasone >400 μg/day
Dry powder inhaler	No use	Some can	Easier to use than MDI
Breath actuated MDI	No use	No use	Over 8 years some can
MDI alone	No use	No use	Good technique essential

Devices and developments

1 Using a large volume spacer device:

  i Essential for those taking more than 800 μg budesonide or beclamethasone, or more than 400 μg fluticasone a day.

  ii Start inhalation as soon as possible after actuating the metered dose inhaler as the drug aerosol rapidly disperses (half life within 10 s).

  iii Single dose at a time. Two rapidly successive actuations can actually reduce the available aerosol by a 'rain' effect, precipitating drug on to the walls of the spacer.

  iv Drug delivery by spacer may be equal to or better than a nebulizer.

2 Turbohalers
  These may deliver twice as much inhaled steroid as an MDI.
  Peak flow required to activate can go as low as 20 l/minute, but amount administered is not consistent.

Controversies in prescribing and management

Prescriptions for asthma have increased by three quarters and GP consultation rate and hospital inpatient episodes doubled from 1985 to 1995. In 1995 the NHS spent £450 million on asthma of all ages, including £380 million on prescriptions.

Steroids

Although recommended by some authorities, a consistent, measurable benefit has not been found in:

1 Initiating treatment with a higher dose, versus a standard dose, of inhaled steroids.
2 Doubling the inhaled dose during colds (becoming standard practice).

Long-term oral steroids now rarely used and seem redundant with more effective inhaled treatment available even if there are concerns over the latter's side effects, namely:

1 Concern about long-term effects of inhaled steroids on the developing lung should restrict use in mild asthmatics, in whom cromoglycate is preferred.
2 Growth impairment: doses greater than 400 μg budesonide or beclamethasone show a short-term effect, but this does not appear to be sustained. Children on higher doses of steroids should have their height monitored.
3 Osteoporosis in adults on prolonged inhaled high dose steroid links with concerns about bone density and mineral accretion in growing children.

β_2-agonists

Almost all biological systems show tolerance to sustained stimulation. A Canadian study of adult asthma deaths implicated *regular* use of β_2-agonists.

- Short-acting β_2-agonists should be given on an 'as required' basis. Long-acting β_2-agonist salmeterol can still be recommended, but care is needed.
- Long-acting β_2-agonist, e.g. salmeterol, may be introduced at step 2 to reduce the need for higher-dose inhaled steroid at step 3.
- Salbutamol syrup in infancy is unlikely to result in the mismatch in ventilation and perfusion found when nebulized β_2-agonist is given.

Cromoglycate

- Efficacy: doubtful under a year old, unless a wheezy ex-prem, and none in acute episodes.
- Oral ketotifen may have a limited place in the preschool child when inhalation prophylaxis is not accepted.

Theophylline

If given i.v. in status asthmaticus, literature review shows it confers no measurable added benefit. Nausea and emesis are significantly increased with its use. Nevertheless, it remains a recommended drug for severe status. Monitor drug levels if given for more than 24 h.

In maintenance therapy it may still be useful, in promoting diaphragmatic contractility, mucociliary clearance, aiding cardiac function, lowering pulmonary artery pressure. Some anti-inflammatory activity has been detected in low dose.

Anti-leucotrienes

A new class of drugs which act by inhibiting 5-lipoxygenase or as leukotriene receptor antagonists. Advantages are oral administration and no significant side effects yet reported, most beneficial in severe asthma, but efficacy only moderate. Their position in stepped management remains to be defined.

Contraindicated at any age

Sedatives, theophylline suppositories. Absorption of the latter is too unpredictable, so giving extra i.v./orally is hazardous.

Usually unhelpful are antihistamines, and antibiotics unless specifically indicated. Still prescribed far too often.

Non-pharmaceutical interventions confirmed as relevant

Avoidance of allergens

Removal of pets, especially cats, and the use of bed covers can reduce symptoms in established asthmatics with positive skin tests.

Audit

Asthma (and diabetes) has been targeted by purchasing authorities in the National Health Service as a means of evaluating and comparing the quality of care of asthma within and between hospitals and general practices.

Multicentre audit of hospital treatment has been hampered by inadequate data in the clinical notes and lack of uniformity of practice between centres.

Hospital audit criteria include

- Child previously seen – in A & E within previous 24 h and/or previous hospital admission in the past 2 weeks (i.e. was treatment inadequate?).
- On admission – recording oxygen saturation, and peak flow rate (PFR) from 7 years old, pulse, respiratory rate, ability to talk, feed (i.e. to assess severity).
- At discharge – were inhaled steroids indicated and commenced, or dose increased and a personalized treatment plan provided (i.e. aim to prevent readmission, and was this admission a failure of prophylaxis?).

Example of optimal audit standards to be applied to general practice

>90% of records to show:

- Trigger factors and family history of atopy.
- PFRs recorded at visits to the GP's office in the past one year.
- Personalized treatment plan on a card if taking inhaled steroid.
- If a bronchodilator is being used twice daily the prescription is changed from cromoglycate to inhaled steroid.

- <20% of children absent from school or missing more than 5 days in 6 months.
- <10% prescribed antibiotics.

Further reading

Ayres J (1994) Asthma and the atmosphere. Leader. *British Medical Journal*, **309**, 619–620

McKenzie S A (1994) Cough – but is it asthma? *Archives of Diseases in Childhood*, **70**, 1–2

McKenzie S A (1994) Aminophylline in the hospital treatment of children with acute asthma. Leader. *British Medical Journal*, **308**, 1384

Silverman M (ed.) (1995) *Childhood asthma and other wheezing disorders*. London: Chapman and Hall

Sporik R. Holgate S T, Cogswell J J (1991) The natural history of asthma in childhood: a birth cohort study. *Archives of Disease in Childhood*, **66**, 1050–1053

Warner J O, Gotz M, Landau L I *et al* (1989) Management of asthma: a consensus statement. *Archives of Disease in Childhood*, **64**, 1065–1979

Warner J O *et al* (1992) Asthma: a follow up statement from an International Paediatric Asthma Consensus Group. *Archives of Disease in Childhood*, **647**, 240–248

ACUTE BRONCHITIS

Definition

Acute inflammation of the trachea and bronchi characterized by:

1 Cough, initially dry, becomes loose in 2–3 days, with sputum usually swallowed. Temperature 37–39°C.
2 Later a few coarse crackles and low pitched wheezes are heard.

Aetiology

Common, usually viral, a feature of measles, occasionally due to *Haemophilus influenzae* and pertussis in the young child, often *Mycoplasma pneumoniae* by school age.

Differential diagnosis

High pitched widespread wheeze is likely to be asthma. Persistent cough beyond 2 weeks is suggestive of segmental collapse or secondary bacterial infection.

Management

1 Cough suppressants: may be harmful, so be cautious.
2 Antibiotics: despite growth of bacteria from throat swabs, and purulent sputum, there is little evidence that antibiotics alter the natural history. Amoxycillin, effective against common secondary bacterial pathogens, is permitted if the cough persists for more than 2 weeks. Failure to respond after a week of antibiotic is an indication to consider further investigation (see chronic cough), unless during a mycoplasma outbreak when erythromycin is the drug of first choice, given for 2–3 weeks.

Recurrent bronchitis

Definition

Recurrent episodes (up to 3–4 per annum) of acute bronchitis, affecting as many as 5% of children, mainly in the first 7 years of life.

Viruses are the primary cause, secondary bronchial irritation from cigarette smoking (active and passive), occasionally dust or fumes.

Differential diagnosis includes asthma, sinusitis, foreign body, bronchiectasis, cystic fibrosis, immune disorders, immotile cilia syndrome, tuberculosis.

In community based studies asthma has frequently been misdiagnosed as bronchitis, with a rewarding improvement in symptoms and school attendance after commencing appropriate therapy.

PNEUMONIAS

Overview of causes, symptoms and signs, investigations, management and prognosis

1   Differentiation of bacterial (10%) from viral (90%), or the common from the esoteric is not possible on clinical grounds.
2   Bronchopneumonia is far commoner in the preschool child than a circumscribed lobar pneumonia.
3   Primary, or secondary to prior infection (e.g. measles, pertussis), aspiration or debilitation.

Symptoms and signs

1   Cough. Usually non-specific. If present in a neonate must be taken seriously.
2   Restless, agitated.
3   Signs: grunting, air hunger and tachypnoea. Cyanosis. Head retracted, flaring of alae nasi, sternal, intercostal and subcostal recession.
4   Complications: unusual – pleural effusions occur in pneumococcal, and pneumothoraces and empyemas in staphylococcal infection.

Investigations

1   Throat swabs are not diagnostic. Better but barely adequate is a cough swab, or sputum via oropharyngeal suction.
2   Blood cultures are often positive in bacterial pneumonias.
3   Immunofluorescent tests for some viral infections (respiratory syncytial virus, influenza etc) allow rapid diagnosis, otherwise culture delays identification for weeks.
4   Traditional antibody tests with a fourfold rise still have a place, e.g. *Mycoplasma pneumoniae*.
5   Tracheal/bronchial aspirate is indicated if an unusual pathogen (e.g. *Pneumocystis carinii*) is suspected, or response to therapy is slow.
6   Leucopenia: total WBC of <5000/mm^3 has a poor prognosis.

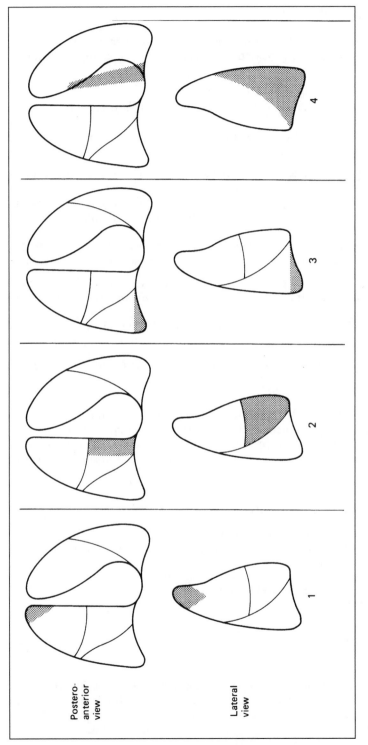

Figure 1.10
Important pneumonic segments not to miss when reviewing postero-anterior X-ray films
1 = Right upper lobe, upper segment
2 = Right middle lobe, medial segment
3 = Right lower lobe, lower segment
4 = Left lower lobe. Look behind the heart

7   Do blood gases if very ill.
8   Chest X-ray (Figure 1.10): may show consolidation before clinical signs are present. Lateral may show unsuspected involvement of the lower lobes. Films should be repeated 3–4 weeks later to ensure resolution.

Management

Observe at home unless toxic, cyanosed, feeding poorly, or parental need for supportive nursing.
   If oral fluid administration causes distress, nasogastric or i.v. fluids must be given to avoid dehydration.

1   Oxygen via a tent (max. oxygen concentration possible 30–40%), mask, nasal catheter or prongs according to age and tolerance.
2   Aspiration of nasopharyngeal secretions. Physiotherapy in the recovery phase; use with care, as excessive handling may tip an ill infant into respiratory failure.
3   Medication: antipyretics + antibiotics are administered according to the most likely bacterial pathogens for age, despite most infections being viral.

   i   <1 year old: flucloxacillin + gentamicin i.v. covers the common pneumococcus, the not unusual *Escherichia coli*, and rare *Staphylococcus aureus*.
   ii   >1 year old: penicillin for pneumococcus while ampicillin also covers *Haemophilus influenzae*. If Legionella is suspected, give erythromycin.

4   Drainage of effusion (pneumococcal) or empyema (staphylococcal).

Prognosis

1   Previously well: good. Resolution of pneumococcal pneumonia 7–10 days, viral and mycoplasma 2–3 weeks, staphylococcal 4+ weeks.
2   Underlying abnormality present (congenital heart disease, immune deficiency, cerebral palsy, etc), especially if already in hospital: slower to respond and a higher mortality.

Failure of pneumonia to resolve

1   Inadequate/inappropriate antibiotic therapy.
2   Pleural effusions (aspirate to dryness, may need a drain) or empyema (surgical decortication).
3   Foreign body (non-radiopaque) requiring bronchoscopy.
4   Cystic fibrosis and immunodeficiency states.
5   Bronchiectasis.

Pneumococcal pneumonia

Epidemiology

1   The cause of 90% of bacterial pneumonias, commonest in 3–8 year olds. Usually sporadic, but an increased risk exists in schools and nurseries after a preceding viral respiratory infection.
2   Bronchopneumonic pattern in infants, lobar at older ages.

Clinical

1 Respiratory: ill child, herpes febrilis on the lips, fine crackles, consolidation.
2 Abdominal distension and ileus, and, with abdominal pain, may mimic acute appendicitis if the right lower lobe (inflammation of the pleura over the diaphragm) is affected.
3 Febrile convulsion, occasionally meningism (especially with right upper lobe) in the preschool child.
4 Associated focal infection, usually limited to otitis media.

Staphylococcus aureus

Infants are usually the age group affected. Uncommon.

Pathophysiology

May seem an ordinary bronchopneumonia until X-rayed. This shows single or multiple cysts full of pus or air or both developing from areas of consolidation. Ball-valve mechanisms operate, tension cysts (pneumatoceles) develop, (sometimes displacing the mediastinum), which may rupture causing pneumothoraces, empyemas and sudden worsening, all within hours.

Clinical

Preceded by staphylococcal skin sepsis contact, or coryzal for up to a week.
  Rapidly become toxic and shocked. Chest involvement is unilateral more than bilateral, right more than left.

Investigations

1 Bacteriology from cough swab, pleural tap, blood culture. (Tracheal aspirate is rarely justified.)
2 Frequent chest X-rays to monitor.
3 Sweat test for cystic fibrosis, screen for immune deficiency.

Differential diagnosis

• Klebsiella pneumonia is similar.
• Foreign body with pulmonary abscess, preceded by an aspiration incident which may have been missed.
• Primary tuberculous pneumonia with cavitation is rarely seen in children in the UK.
• X-ray may be confused with a diaphragmatic hernia.

Management

1 Antistaphylococcal drugs for 4+ weeks.
2 Surgical drainage of empyema.

3   Needling and underwater drainage for gross obstructive distension/ pneumothorax.

Prognosis

Prognosis is good if the condition is recognized early. Surprisingly the chest X-ray returns to normal within 2–3 months.

Haemophilus influenzae

Slower onset than pneumococcal, otherwise similar presentation.

   Pyogenic complications are common: septicaemia, cellulitis, septic arthritis, pericarditis, empyema, meningitis.

Mycoplasma pneumoniae

Usually symptomatic in the 5–15 year old age group. Incubation 2–3 weeks, often running in families.

Clinical

Mild respiratory symptoms for days or weeks, not very ill with diffuse signs on X-ray more marked than clinically apparent. Cough productive of mucoid or even blood tinged sputum. Chest pain not uncommon. Occasionally may have a high swinging temperature and be quite toxic. Clinical associations: maculopapular rashes, erythema nodosum, meningitis, myringitis bullosa. McLeod syndrome is a late complication.

Investigation

Cold agglutinins are positive in half of the patients. Specific antibody test required for accurate diagnosis.

Management

Erythromycin for 2–3 weeks may be effective.

Adenovirus

Types 3, 7, 21. Especially severe in young children.

   Chronic sequelae, which are rare: hyperinflation, wheeze, recurrent infection and atelectasis due to obliterating bronchiolitis, pulmonary fibrosis, and bronchiectasis.

Chlamydia trachomatis

Uncommon. Acquired during delivery from mother's genital tract, presenting at 4–15 weeks old.

Pertussis-like cough, tachypnoea, fine crackles.

50% have conjunctivitis and/or otitis media.

Interstitial infiltrates and hyperinflation on chest X-ray, mild eosinophilia in the blood. Cultures are needed as antibody tests are unreliable. Erythromycin for 2–3 weeks, to both parents as well as the infant, to prevent recurrence. Chronic cough may persist for weeks.

Pneumocystis carinii

Immune deficiency disorders, primary or secondary, are necessary for infection by this protozoan of low virulence.

Features include dry cough, tachypnoea, cyanosis with variable fever, little on auscultation compared with extensive X-ray changes of infiltrates and a ground glass appearance.

Diagnosis: pneumocystis cysts on lung biopsy or bronchoscopy in small children. Cough induced by hypertonic saline inhalation is productive of cysts in >50% of young adults with AIDS and is less hazardous.

Prognosis

Death if untreated or diagnosis excessively delayed. Give co-trimoxazole (full course, then alternate days for prophylaxis), or pentamidine.

ACUTE RESPIRATORY FAILURE

Definition

Elevated P_{CO_2} during an acute illness (>7 kPa or 49 mmHg, 5.6 kPa or 40 mmHg in asthma). Levels of 8–9 kPa (56–63 mmHg) are consistent with the need for mechanical ventilation.

Low Pa_{O_2} in air is common.

Pathophysiology

See introduction to the chapter on pages 5–7.

Clinical signs are often *more* important than gases: cyanosis/extreme pallor, severe respiratory distress, decreased respiratory effort, 'silent' chest, confused, coma, hypotonia, exhaustion, plus signs from any underlying disease process.

Beware 'healthy' pink vasodilated drowsy child in oxygen rich atmosphere sinking into CO_2 narcosis.

Causes

1 Previously well

   i   Accidents: trauma, burns, drowning, poisoning, foreign body.
   ii Upper airway obstruction: stridor (see causes), tonsillar hypertrophy.
   iii Lower respiratory tract: asthma, bronchiolitis, pneumonia.
   iv CNS abnormality: encephalitis, seizures, polyneuritis.
   v   Septicaemia, metabolic disorders.

2 Underlying abnormality

   i   Cystic fibrosis.
   ii Scoliosis (severe) with infection, or postoperatively.
   iii Congenital heart disease.
   iv Neuromuscular diseases, e.g. Duchenne muscular dystrophy, myasthenia.

Management

1 Early respiratory failure: treat the underlying condition vigorously. Minimal handling.
2 Established respiratory failure: first consider if an underlying abnormality precludes treatment, e.g. advanced cystic fibrosis, Werdnig–Hoffman disease.

Practical aspects of intubation

1 Bag and mask with 100% oxygen.
2 Endotracheal intubation:

   i   Uncuffed tube if under 8 years old.
   ii Tube size not too tight, to avoid pressure necrosis, or too small a diameter with increased airway resistance. Formula = (age/4) +4 = size in mm.
   iii Change to nasoendotracheal intubation, once the airway is controlled, if prolonged support for days is likely.
       Always check:

       a. Air entry lest you are only ventilating the right main bronchus.
       b. Chest X-ray to confirm the tube position (shorten if necessary).

3 Humidification and frequent suction of the tube to prevent blockage.
4 Arm restraints to prevent the child extubating himself. With judicious sedation they may be removed later.
5 Establish an arterial line, repeat blood gases 4–6 hourly, adjust ventilator settings for normalization of gases. Continuous positive airway pressure helps avoid alveolar collapse.
6 As improvement occurs, reduce pressures, oxygen, and rate, in that order.
   Fluids i.v. 0.18% saline + 4.3% dextrose, with added potassium.

Volume according to weight and condition: e.g. increased in asthma, reduced if a danger of cerebral oedema due to asphyxia or inappropriate antidiuretic hormone release secondary to stress.

CYSTIC FIBROSIS (CF)

Definition

Characterized by malabsorption and failure to thrive due to exocrine pancreatic insufficiency and chronic suppurative lung disease in 80–90%, meconium ileus in 17% of affected newborns, obstructive biliary tract disease in 15%, diabetes mellitus in 20% of adults and azoospermia in >90% of affected men. Inherited in an AR pattern, antenatal diagnosis is possible in informative families.

Incidence

One in 2000 Caucasians, the commonest lethal inherited disorder, carried by 1 in 25 of the population. The incidence is much lower in other races. In the USA 30 000 affected.

Size of the problem

Two hundred and fifty new CF children born annually in the UK; 80% are now expected to survive to adult life.

Genetic basis for CF and prenatal diagnosis

The gene on chromosome 7 produces an abnormal CF transport protein, 'cystic fibrosis transmembrane conductance regulator' (CFTR), in the cell membrane. Up to 75% of UK Caucasian children may have the same mutation (delta F508) so their families are informative using DNA probes; 120 affected fetuses could be identified annually in the UK.

Chorionic villous biopsy accuracy of prediction is 95% in the first trimester. Low intestinal alkaline phosphatase in amniotic fluid in the second trimester will correctly predict 90% of fetuses homozygous for CF where the DNA probe pattern proves uninformative.

Pathophysiology

The metabolic defect lies in the CFTR, with reduced ATP binding and defective chloride ion transport.

Action of CFTR: controls the opening and closing of the chloride channel. Absence of CFTR is thus responsible for the increase in sweat chloride and sodium.

The mucus gland secretions are more sticky than usual, blocking:

1   Pancreatic ducts, which dilate and become cystic; autodigestion, fibrosis and calcification follow. Digestive enzymes and bicarbonate secretion are severely reduced.

2   Bronchioles. In the respiratory tract the serous layer between the surface of the cell and the mucus blanket supported on the tips of the cilia contains less water and electrolytes than normal, and the secretions become viscous. This prevents the normal beating of the cilia thus reducing mucociliary clearance. Response to infection tends to produce even more tenacious mucus, further reducing mucociliary clearance. Repeated infection results, causing more mucus production, obstruction, fibrosis and bronchiectasis, in a vicious cycle. Progressive respiratory failure leads to cor pulmonale.

3   Liver causing focal biliary cirrhosis; also salivary glands, and vas deferens obstruction resulting in sterile males.

- Variability in severity of pancreatic insufficiency, bronchial infection and lung damage are determined by the level of gene expression and function of CFTR. Pancreatic exocrine insufficiency is greater in homozygous ΔF508 than in other mutations, and respiratory deterioration tends to occur earlier.

Factors in lower respiratory infection in CF

1   Cross infection. Risk of the spread of *Pseudomonas aeruginosa*, and increasingly *Burkholderia* (previously *Pseudomonas*) *cepacia*, which has a high mortality, when CF sufferers meet.

2   Absence of CFTR results in impaired mucociliary function and epithelial integrity. Infection begins with staphylococci and *Haemophilus*, later *Pseudomonas* (Ps) colonization. A change in these Ps colonies, from smooth to mucoid alginate producing, heralds progressive lung injury. This alginate layer reduces penetration of antibiotics and neutrophils. Antibodies then develop in excess (high IgG_2 and IgG_3 levels have a worse prognosis), form immune complexes activating macrophages into an inflammatory reaction. Leukotrienes (chemotaxins) are released from macrophages and neutrophils in response to *Ps. aeruginosa*, intensifying the activity.

3   Inflammatory response persists. Neutrophils release enzymes, e.g. elastase, and generate oxygen metabolites, e.g. hydrogen peroxide, damaging elastin and other lung tissue proteins. Cytokines are liberated, and may also cause severe weight loss.

We can conclude:

- CF lung inflammation is neutrophil dominated.
- Control of the inflammatory response could limit lung damage.

4   Excess DNA increases sputum viscosity. The excess DNA is from the breakdown of large numbers of polymorphs and damaged cells.

Therapeutic interventions arising:

1   Segregation of *Burkholderia cepacia* cases to reduce cross infection.

2   i   Early continuous antibiotic treatment to inhibit or delay chronic infection and subsequent lung damage – trials are inconclusive at present.
     ii   Gene therapy: transfection to the lungs of CF sufferers with viruses

engineered to contain normal CFTR copy DNA. Early trials in adults have been promising. The ultimate hoped for cure for CF.

3   Anti-inflammatory medication. Initial trials show they curb lung damage. Not yet in routine clinical use.

   i   Inhaled steroid. Initiate early, in high dose? Placebo controlled study not yet done; oral was trialed but serious late steroid side effects resulted (growth failure, cataracts).
   ii Non-steroidal anti-inflammatories: ibuprofen, early trial is promising.

4   DNase as an aerolysed enzyme has a beneficial effect on viscosity and mucociliary clearance.

Clinical presentation

Initial presentation:
   Meconium ileus 17%.
   Malabsorption 30%.
   Chest infection 50%.

By age

1   Neonatal: meconium ileus. Some perforate causing peritonitis, and need a temporary ileostomy.
2   Infancy (common)

   i   Recurrent chest infection. Finger clubbing follows later.
   ii Failure to thrive, steatorrhoea.
   iii Developmental delay caused by (i) and (ii).

3   Toddler/child, above plus

   i   Rectal prolapse in 20%.
   ii Heat stroke.

4   Older child, above plus

   i   Asthma in 20%, allergic aspergillosis 10%.
   ii Meconium ileus equivalent in 20% = recurrent colicky abdominal pain, distension, constipation, a mass of impacted faeces in the right iliac fossa. Rarely, complete obstruction from volvulus or intussusception (1%) occurs.
   iii Sinusitis 90%, nasal polyps 10%.

5   Adolescence, above plus

   i   Delayed puberty with short stature is very common.
   ii Respiratory function deteriorates markedly in females. Haemoptysis, repeated pneumothorax in young adults.
   iii Liver cirrhosis is commonly subclinical – portal hypertension 10%, with bleeding oesophageal varicies 1%. Gallstones in the teens in 10%. Pancreatitis rare.
   iv Diabetes mellitus in 10–40%, from 10 years of age.

v Arthritis: hypertrophic pulmonary osteoarthropathy 10%, intermittent polyarthropathy occasionally.

vi Infertility. Males: 97% affected due to atretic vas deferens and epididymus. Females are subfertile due to abnormal cervical mucus.

Consider CF in the following situations

1 Respiratory symptoms

- After a second pneumonia in infancy (or first if staphylococcal).
- Frequent bronchitis (not asthma) with paroxysmal cough.
- Hyperinflated, pigeon chest, intercostal recession and Harrison's sulci are later signs.
- Pseudomonas (mucoid strain) chest infection.
- Staphylococcal pneumonia.

2 Growth and bowel symptoms

- Meconium ileus, meconium plug syndrome.
- Failure to thrive (progressing to gross wasting), voracious appetite, with offensive loose, frequent, small stools which later become bulky, putty coloured, oily.
- Rectal prolapse.

3 Family history and asymptomatic

Table 1.8 Differential diagnosis of recurrent wheeze

---

1 Reactive airways
   Asthma (atopic family history, thriving, though in severe asthma CF must be excluded).
   Wheezy baby syndrome often affects chubby (not wasted) infants.
   Extrinsic allergic alveolitis will give a history of exposure.
2 Infective
   Post pertussis, vomiting prominent.
   Loeffler's syndrome, e.g. *Toxocara canis*, drugs.
3 Mechanical
   Recurrent aspiration due to hiatal hernia.
   Foreign body, compression from glands, tumours, aberrant vessels.
   Congenital lung abnormality: bronchogenic cyst, sequestrated lobe, lobar emphysema, cystic adenomatous malformation.
4 Cardiac failure
5 Genetic and acquired impaired respiratory tract defence
   Cystic fibrosis.
   Immune deficiency: unusual organisms may be grown.
   Immotile cilia syndrome, including Kartegener's syndrome: (AR, reduced cilial function due to abnormal cilial structure causes sinusitis, serous otitis, bronchiectasis, infertility as sperm are immotile, situs inversus in 50%).

Diagnosis of cystic fibrosis

1   Sweat test

   i Sweat sodium of >70 mmol/kg by pilocarpine iontophoresis, weight of sweat >100 mg, on two occasions, is necessary for confirmation of CF. Repeat if >50 mmol/kg.

  ii Osmolality of the sweat obtained >220 mmol/kg, using special collection equipment, has low errors compared with (i), the traditional 'gold standard' test.

2 Screening: serum immunoreactive trypsin (IRT) is raised × 10 normal in the CF newborn. The use of human trypsinogen monoclonal antibody (HTMAB) has improved the accuracy of IRT assay. Guthrie card blood spot is used. Confirm with a sweat test after 1–2 months of age.

3 Genetic studies:

   i Gene site on chromosome 7 is identifiable in 75% from RFLPs.

  ii Antenatal diagnosis by chorionic biopsy, or estimation of microvillar enzymes in the uninformative families.

General management

An annual assessment process has been introduced in many CF clinics at which a planned review of all aspects is considered, not in an opportunistic random fashion. At this visit the topics include: present status, review of events in the past year, microbiology for sputum culture, aspergillus precipitins, lung function, chest X-ray with Chrispin-Norman or other scoring system, blood count and liver function tests, blood sugar and urine for glucose, reviews by physiotherapist, dietician, psychosocial review, and medical assessment.

Prognosis for survival is improved by attending or sharing care with specialist CF treatment centres.

Respiratory management

Encourage vigorous daily exercise; use cromoglycate or β-agonists for any exercise induced wheeze.

1 *Physiotherapy*

Passive postural drainage, percussion (autogenic or by parent), forced expiration techniques (huffing), or use of a device (Flutter) for 10–15 minutes, 2–4 times daily, proportional to sputum production and symptoms. Hypertonic saline (3–5%) inhalation aids coughing. Adolescents often need supervision to keep this up.

2 *Antibiotics*

  a. Acute infection: as sputum culture and sensitivities indicate, for 2–3 weeks. In infancy: flucloxacillin in case of *Staphylococcus aureus*.

     Later: *Pseudomonas* species appear, and cannot be completely eliminated, but respond to a combination of i.v. aminoglycoside (monitor blood levels, often need more) and ureidopenicillin or third generation cephalosporin. Oral ciprofloxacin is a good cheap alternative, despite emerging resistance and reservations about it causing arthropathy in young animals. Arthropathy occurs in 7–8% of CF children but is not increased following exposure to ciprofloxacin.

    b. More continuous treatment for increased sputum production and weight loss. Frequent courses inevitably produce resistant strains. *Haemophilus influenzae* causes some exacerbations. Strict infection control and cohorting outpatient/ward contact minimizes spread of resistant bacteria.

    c. Prevention/reduction in lung damage.
Controversy continues concerning its efficacy.

      Infancy: studies inconclusive, whether to give antistaphylococcal drugs either as clinically indicated, or continuously for the first 5 years, or possibly for life. Worries about emerging resistant strains.

      Late, once colonized by pseudomonas: i.v. antipseudomonal drugs at regular 3 monthly intervals, may be self-administered at home via a subcutaneously implanted reservoir.

3   *Inhaled therapy*
Of proven usefulness in the following situations:

    a. To improve the removal of secretions: hypertonic saline, salbutamol, acetyl cysteine before physiotherapy.

    b. Continued deterioration or frequent hospital admissions, give home nebulized gentamicin, or tobramycin, + carbenicillin 2 × daily.

    c. Bronchospasm as shown by 10% improvement following inhaled β_2-agonist. Aim: bronchodilatation and reduction of inflammatory oedema – give salbutamol, budesonide or betamethasone, or cromoglycate.

    d. Recombinant human DNase (rhDNase) 2.5 mg b.d. for moderate CF with chronic endobronchial bacterial infection with purulent secretions and obstructive pattern of lung function. Trials show a significant reduction in the risk of respiratory infection needing i.v. antibiotics. Cost is high (£4000 for 6 months).

4   *Monitor progress by*

    a. Regular (monthly) sputum cultures for organisms and sensitivity patterns.

    b. Chest X-ray (6 monthly). Changes begin in the upper zones.

    c. Assess lung function 6 monthly from 5 years old: FEV_1, FVC, and FEV_1/FVC ratio follow an obstructive airways pattern, influenced by antibiotics, physiotherapy, and diet.

      Where appropriate, monitoring for complications of advanced disease:
Monitor oxygen to avoid CO_2 narcosis; brown sputum is suggestive of *Aspergillus fumigatus*; heart failure occurs due to cor pulmonale.

5   *Immunization*
Pertussis, measles; annual influenza vaccination from 4 years old.

Nutritional management

Ninety per cent have pancreatic insufficiency. Maintaining adequate weight is a key factor in long-term survival.

    Many children are small for age and enter puberty 2 years late. Height and weight must be regularly charted.

Steatorrhoea occurs when 90% of pancreatic function is lost. Assess by fat balance over 3 days; >10% loss in faeces is abnormal. A full fat diet is recommended, for in the past fat avoidance caused unnecessary subnutrition, and possibly contributed to a poorer prognosis.

Nutritional requirements 110–150% of recommended daily allowances.

Nutritional advances

Improved nutrition results in better growth and prolonged survival. Reasons:

- Malnutrition impairs muscle function, ventilatory drive and decreased exercise tolerance, and ultimately immune response to infection.
- Increased energy requirements at rest of 9–30% (increased work of breathing, infection, enteral feeds, salbutamol).
- Faecal energy losses are 3 times normal.
- Urinary losses, as glycosuria if diabetes develops.
- Sputum losses can comprise 1–5% of energy intake.
- Salt depletion in infancy impairs growth.

Factors militating against adequate intake

- Reduced appetite due to abdominal pain and vomiting from distal ileus obstruction syndrome, infection, cough, reflux oesophagitis.
- Media preoccupations with 'healthy eating' (low fat, low sugar diet) and the cult of thinness.
- Feeding problems especially toddlers: food fads, dislike of fatty foods.
- Finance.

Nutritional prescriptions

1 Pancreatic enzyme replacement:
   Revised recommendations from the Committee on Safety of Medicines:
   Infants 2–4000 u lipase per 12 ml feed, or 1/2 capsule ordinary strength lipase (average strength 5–8000 units) per breast feed.
   Under 4 years start with 1000 u lipase/kg/meal.
   Older children 500 u lipase/kg/meal to a maximum of 2500 u/kg/meal. Snacks, usually ⅓–½ of the meal dose.
   Excess acidity inactivates these enzyme preparations; add bicarbonate or H_2-receptor antagonist if steatorrhoea, excessive flatus, or abdominal pain persist.
2 Vitamins:
   Prescribe twice the normal requirements of water (B,C) and fat soluble (A,D,E,K) vitamins as daily Abidec, Ketovite tabs and liquid. Vitamin E and K are given separately.
3 Sodium supplements in hot weather.

Management of the non-thriving CF child

In the presence of weight loss or clinical deterioration use the following steps:

1 Optimize respiratory management: antibiotics, physiotherapy, regular exercise, DNAse, frequent monitoring by the CF team, in the clinic and home.

2   Reduce calorie losses by careful attention to dosage of enzymes (avoiding high dose preparations, see below), and checking the product is fresh, as lipase activity declines. A fat balance <85% may indicate the addition of an H_2-receptor antagonist or misoprostol to reduce gastric acidity which denatures the lipase.

3   Check intake: behavioural? Avoid feeding battles, enlist psychological help.

4   Ensure adequate calories with appropriate food supplements, e.g. milk shakes containing 1–1.5 kcal/ml, 4–6 g protein/100 ml and glucose polymers 1.8–4 kcal/ml.

5   Indications for enteral feeds (nasogastric/gastrostomy), required in about 5% of CF:

   i   If appetite remains poor, feeling ill, depressed, breathless.

   ii <85% of weight for height or no weight gain for 3–6 months.

   Give as overnight feeds, 40–50% of total requirements. Hyperglycaemia can be a problem requiring insulin in 30%.

6   Consider complications, e.g. distal ileus obstruction syndrome, diabetes mellitus, cirrhosis. Crohn's and coeliac disease may be more common in CF.

Home care intensification

Home intravenous antibiotic/alimentation. Used in the more advanced case, when weight loss predicts serious deterioration.
   Rationale:

   a. Reduction in hospitalization, its duration and frequency, hence costs and hospital cross infection.
   b. Less disruption and hospital dependency for the family.
   c. Continuity of schooling/employment.

Emotional support

This includes the whole family. Guilt feelings in the parents, the demanding daily schedule of treatment and its rejection, delayed puberty and adolescent rebellion, depression, the death of a CF friend, and career guidance, all require some anticipation and an established network of support.

Transplant

Heart–lung and liver transplants for a selected few is a final treatment option.

Controversy in management

Colonic stricture formation and high dose pancreatic enzyme administration

Up to April 1994, 14 children were reported. Their intake of proteases and lipases was twice that of controls, using preparations containing lipase 22–25 000 units.

   Hypothesis of causation: rapid transit of ingested enzymes not broken down in the small intestine delivers them, still active, to the colon, an area not designed to cope with this part of the digestive process.

Problems in transfer of adolescent CF patients to an adult clinic

Age at transfer 15–17 years, delay often indicated due to emotional and sexual immaturity for age.

The patient is often still in the throes of adolescent rebellion with problems of compliance and emotional dependency.

The parents tend to be overprotective, inhibiting social skills development and independence.

Paediatric team may have strong emotional links with the patient from infancy onwards, or perceive adult care as fragmented, maybe a respiratory physician alone, unable to respond appropriately to the challenges of adolescents.

The handover should be formal, in a joint clinic setting with both paediatric and adult teams (including nurses, physiotherapists, dieticians, social worker) and the parents present.

Prognosis

Median age of survival is 25 years, 80% reaching adult life in the best treatment centres. Specialist adult CF clinics have extended the length and quality of survival into the 30–40 year age bracket.

Nutritional factors: stunting leads to a higher mortality. Pubertal females have a high rate of rapid deterioration, cause unknown.

Sedentary/professional occupations are most suitable, and unemployment is little higher than the rest of the population.

Presymptomatic diagnosis of CF by neonatal screening using IRT may further alter the natural history by earlier treatment.

Identification of the CFTR gene sequence makes DNA replacement therapy possible. (See Leader. (1990) Cystic fibrosis: prospects for screening and therapy, *Lancet*, i, 79–80.)

Further reading

David T J (1990) Cystic fibrosis. *Archives of Disease in Childhood*, **65**, 152–157

Koch C, Hoiby N (1995) Pathogenesis of respiratory disease in cystic fibrosis. In *Recent Advances in Paediatrics 13*, (ed. T.J. David). Edinburgh: Churchill Livingstone p 29–44

MacDonald A (1996) Nutritional management of cystic fibrosis. *Archives of Disease in Childhood*, **74**, 81–87

Ramsay B W (1996) Management of pulmonary disease in patients with cystic fibrosis. *New England Journal of Medicine*, **335**, 179–188

Smyth R L, van Velzen D, Smyth A R *et al* (1994) Strictures of ascending colon in cystic fibrosis and high-strength pancreatic enzymes. *Lancet*, i, 85–86

TUBERCULOSIS (TB)

Aetiology

Mycobacterium tuberculosis is transmitted from an adult with caseating disease. Rarely it is spread transplacentally by seeding amniotic fluid. Bovine TB eradicated from the UK.

Malnutrition, measles and immune deficiency increase susceptibility. Dual infection with HIV is an increasing concern worldwide.

Childhood notifications in the UK

Represent 5% of all new TB cases. Almost half are Asian children. The 1983 Medical Research Council survey rate was 5 per 100 000, (2.4 Caucasian, 17 West Indian, 40 Asian) and 25 times higher if born abroad.

Primary lesion in the lung in 75% (higher in Asians), extrapulmonary 25%.

Adult household contact in 80%, with an infection risk of 10% if the adult is sputum positive, 0.5% (non-Asian) to 3% (Asian) if sputum negative.

Pathology

1   Bacilli ingested by macrophages which activate T lymphocytes. Only 1 in 10 of those infected develop disease, the highest risk being in the first 1–2 years after infection.
2   Delayed hypersensitivity reaction (basis of the Mantoux text) after an incubation period of 2–10 weeks, causing massive local tissue reaction = caseation = the body's attempt to seal off the infection.
3   In the brain, bursting of a tuberculoma seeded by miliary spread causes a similar severe inflammatory reaction, then thick gelatinous exudate which gums up the CSF pathways (hydrocephalus), compresses the cranial nerves and obstructs vessels causing infarcts and swelling.
4   Calcification follows over about 6 months.

Timing of presentation after exposure

1   Hypersensitivity phenomena in 2–10 weeks.
2   Miliary TB and meningitis within 3 months.
3   Pleural effusion and segmental lesions (see below) 3–12 months.
4   Bronchopneumonia, focal infection of other organs 1–5+ years.
5   Post-primary TB 3+ years.

Clinical

1   Hypersensitivity.

    Asymptomatic or with fever for 2–3 weeks, weight loss, general malaise; occasionally phlyctenular conjunctivitis, erythema nodosum, rarely pleural effusion (usually sterile, may clot on standing, containing lymphocytes, occurs in over 5 year olds).

2   Pulmonary TB (75%).

    i   Primary focus with enlargement of hilar lymph glands = primary complex. Heals with calcification.
    ii Mediastinal lymph node involvement with brassy cough (pertussis like), rapid and laboured breathing. Resultant effects:

        a.   Gland enlarges, compressing bronchi, causing segmental collapse, or hyperinflation if a 'ball valve' effect occurs.

b. Contiguous spread of infection into bronchi by erosion and perforation → consolidation + hypersensitivity reaction = 'epituberculosis'. In older children it predominates in the upper lobes; middle and lower lobes in the younger age group.

iii X-ray changes occur after 3 months (Figure 1.11). Findings on presentation:

Pulmonary shadowing (miliary or pneumonic)	45%
Mediastinal lymphadenopathy	38%
Effusion only	4%
Lymph nodes and effusion	3%
Normal X-ray	10%

3 Extrapulmonary sites (25%).
'Cold abscess' in the neck (scrofula), overlying skin of red or purplish hue, usually due to bovine TB.
4 Miliary spread and tuberculous meningitis result if a lymph gland erodes into a blood vessel (i.e. post primary TB).
Commonest age and most at risk are children aged less than 3 years old. Peak onset is 1–6 months after a primary infection.
Findings:

i Fever, anorexia, weight loss.
ii Respiratory: cough, tachypnoea, pneumonia, with 'snow storm' appearance of generalized mottling on X-ray.
iii Abdomen: distended by hepatosplenomegaly.

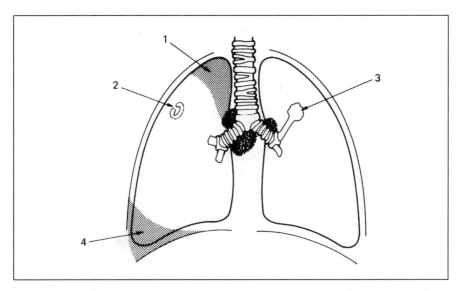

Figure 1.11 Typical changes associated with the primary complex to look for on chest X-ray
1. RUL collapse due to mediastinal nodes
2. Nodular lesion of calcified primary complex
3. Cavitation
4. Effusion/empyema

iv CNS: progressive lethargy, coma, opisthotonus, convulsions; choroidal
tubercles in 50%; CSF shows lymphocytosis, low glucose, raised
protein, occasional acid fast bacilli.

5 Abdominal TB from bovine source (immigrant from underdeveloped
country) or swallowing respiratory tract secretions. Rarely symptomatic,
when an ulcerative colitis picture is seen, or tuberculous peritonitis with
ascites or matted guts.

Reactivation: adult or chronic TB

Rare in childhood.
Pulmonary caseation and cavitation in adolescents. Kidneys at 3 years, bones
and joints (knee, hip, spine) 5 years after primary infection.

Investigation

1 Mantoux, ESR; X-ray of chest, spine or long bone if affected; early
morning gastric washings × 3 for acid fast bacilli and culture (takes 6
weeks). Culture positive 20% in lymph node and pulmonary infection,
50% in meningeal infection. NB: Mantoux may be negative in severe
disease, and in up to 40% with TB meningitis.
2 In lymphadenopathy, bone and joint disease: biopsy or aspirate for
histology and culture.
3 Bone marrow or liver aspirate is helpful in diagnosing miliary spread.
4 In meningitis obtain CSF, consider CT of the head to identify hydrocephalus and tuberculomas.

New, experimental diagnostic aids include enzyme linked immunosorbent
assay of *M. tuberculosis* antigen and DNA probes of mycobacterial RNA.
Rapid confirmation with great accuracy is claimed.

Differential diagnosis includes:

1 Atypical mycobacterial *Mycobacterium avium intracellulare* (MAI):
presentation commonly as submandibular and cervical lymphadenitis.
HIV associated.
   The Mantoux reaction with PPD is 5–12 mm. Biopsy and culture
needed. Standard antituberculous drugs are usually ineffective, but surgical removal is usually curative.
2 Sarcoid: rare in children, commoner in adolescents. Non-caseating granu-
loma found in affected lymph gland or on Kveim test (rarely done).
Characterized by breathlessness and dry cough. Uveitis and erythema
nodosum may be associated. Hilar lymphadenopathy, possibly with
widespread infiltrates. Steroids are only indicated for uveitis.

Treatment of TB (Table 1.9)

1 Active disease (notifiable)

Promptly commence on the basis of a positive Mantoux, or negative but
suspicious results in an ill, febrile child from a high risk background.

Table 1.9 First line antituberculous drug regimens and their duration

Initial phase (in months as n/12)		Continuation phase	Months of drugs
1 Active disease any site:*	R I P for 2/12	R I for 4/12	Total 6/12
	or R I for 2/12	R I for 7/12	Total 9/12
2 Chemoprophylaxis	I for 6/12		Total 6/12
	R I for 3/12		Total 3/12

*Treat meningitis for 1 year minimum
R = rifampicin 10–20 mg/kg/day (colours urine red, warn parents; major side effect hepatitis – substitute with ethambutol)
I = isoniazid 10 mg/kg/day (pyridoxine is unnecessary unless cachectic as peripheral neuritis is not found in children)
P = pyrazinamide 35 mg/kg/day (initial facial flushing, rash, nausea, arthralgia, hepatitis)

Second line drugs for children:

  i Ethambutol 10–15 mg/kg/day usually only until sensitivity of organism is established, i.e. the first 2 months (but the risk of optic neuritis, requiring ophthalmic supervision, makes it unsuitable for young children).

  ii Streptomycin for tuberculous meningitis in the first 2–3 months.

  iii Prednisolone lowers raised intracranial pressure, may help in hilar compression, pericarditis, pleural effusion, miliary disease, and is given for 4–8 weeks.

Drug resistance: Caucasians very rare, up to 10% in Asians. To minimize this, 2 or 3 drugs are always given together in active disease.
Compliance must be checked regularly.
Cure is about 95% on the primary course of chemotherapy. Failure, relapse, or toxicity in the remainder will respond to an altered regimen.
Assess progress with serial ESR, X-rays, weight gain, clinical signs.

2   Chemotherapy (does not require notification)

  i Heaf positive, normal ESR and chest X-ray, give if:
No previous BCG and grade 2–4.
Previous BCG and grade 3–4.

  ii Heaf/Mantoux negative child, recently exposed to known infectious adult.

  iii Previously treated or has become immunosuppressed, e.g. from steroids/chemotherapy, AIDS.

  iv Neonate of infected mother: continue breast feeding. Isoniazid for 3 months then check X-ray and Mantoux to determine whether to continue medication. In the UK it is policy to give BCG if negative, not so in the USA.

Contact tracing   Delay in diagnosis is a hazard for contacts of the index case, and a large number of children may be infected before action is taken (Figure 1.12).

Prognosis

Excellent with treatment; rarely is there residual lung scarring, or bronchiectasis.

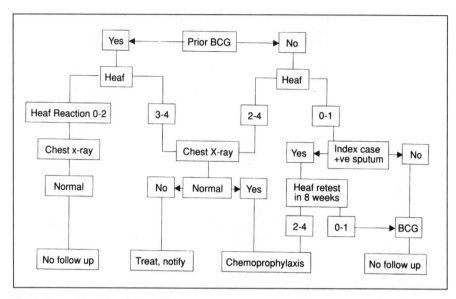

Figure 1.12   Algorithm for TB contact cases

Most deaths occur in infancy and adolescence, which directs preventive strategy at these age groups.

Early diagnosis is critical in TB meningitis to avoid the feared complications (hydrocephalus, blindness, deafness, cerebral palsy, death).

Prevention

1   Screen all new immigrants from India and other developing countries. Identifies those needing treatment, chemoprophylaxis or BCG.
2   Bacille Calmette-Guérin (BCG) is given:

   i   At birth: almost 100% protection against TB meningitis and miliary TB in under 2 year olds. Recommended for those of African and Asian origin. Caucasian babies should also be offered it in areas with a high Afro-Asian immigrant mix. Revaccination in adolescence is desirable.
   ii Adolescence: 75% protected for at least 10 years. Routine testing of all children with Tine test or Heaf test at 13 years identifies those at risk. If the incidence of TB continues to fall, and HIV associated TB is contained, routine vaccination may be withdrawn.

NB: TB is notifiable to the local Medical Officer of Environmental Health (England and Wales), so that potential contacts are traced and assessed.

Further reading

Leader (1990) Perinatal prophylaxis of tuberculosis. *Lancet*, ii, 1479–1480
Leader (1988) Childhood tuberculosis in Britain. *British Medical Journal*, **297**, 1147–1148

Medical Research Council Tuberculosis and Chest Diseases Unit (1989) *Archives of Disease in Childhood*, **64**, 1004–1012

Snider D E, Rieder H L, Combs D, Bloch A B, Hayden C H, Smith M H D (1988) Tuberculosis in children. *Pediatric Infectious Disease Journal*, **7**, 271–278

Starke J R (1988) Modern approach to the diagnosis and management of tuberculosis in children. *Pediatric Clinics of North America*, **35**, 441–464

IMMUNE RELATED DISORDERS AFFECTING THE LUNGS (ALL RARE)

1 Idiopathic interstitial pneumonitis

Macrophages accumulate in the interstitium. Alveolar epithelial hyperplasia follows, desquamating into the alveoli, blocking them. The result is restrictive lung disease with impaired CO diffusion on testing.

Clinical

Breathless, dry cough, tired, weight loss. Cyanosis, finger clubbing and fine crackles on auscultation.

Investigations

Ground glass lung fields on X-ray. Hypoxia, hypocapnia leading to hypercapnia later.

Management

Steroids or antimetabolites may help, otherwise prognosis is poor.

2 Autoimmune

Complicating rheumatoid arthritis, systemic lupus erythematosus, as part of Goodpasture's syndrome and other connective tissue disorders. An interstitial pneumonitis with findings similar to the idiopathic variety, but usually more responsive to steroids and antimetabolites.

3 Pulmonary haemosiderosis

Bleeding into the lungs, cause usually idiopathic, occasionally seen in cows' milk protein intolerance and Goodpasture's syndrome.

Clinical

Fever, cough, wheeze and intra-alveolar haemorrhage resulting in anaemia and rusty sputum.

Investigations

Chest X-ray varies from minor areas of consolidation that clear within a week to extensive bilateral mottling. Repeated bleeds cause interstitial opaque nodules.

Gastric aspirate contains haemosiderin laden macrophages.

Management

Transfusion, steroids, iron. Trial of cows' milk avoidance. May respond to antimetabolites.

Further reading

Textbooks:

Dinwiddie R (1990) *The Diagnosis and Management of Paediatric Respiratory Disease.* Edinburgh: Churchill Livingstone
Phelan P D, Landau L I, Olinsky A. (1990) *Respiratory Illness in Children* 3rd edn. Oxford: Blackwell Scientific

Chapter 2

Cardiology update, including cardiorespiratory arrest and hypotension*

CARDIOLOGY

Congenital heart disease is primarily structural and is a result of embryonic maldevelopment of the heart.

Embryology

The cardiovascular system is the first system to function in the embryo. By the end of the fifth week the heart has developed from two endocardial heart tubes into a complex four chambered organ, which is completed by week eight. The embryological basis of the common heart defects will be shown.

Dextrocardia

This occurs when the the tube bends to the left instead of the right.

- Defects are common if it is *isolated* and probably no greater than normal in the presence of situs inversus. The association with ciliary dyskinesia (Kartagener syndrome = situs inversus, chronic sinusitis, nasal polyps, bronchiectasis, male infertility) occurs in 15–25%.

Atrial septal defect (ASD)

Divided into primum and secundum ASDs.

Primum ASD

A thin crescent-shaped membrane grows from the roof of the atrium towards the atrioventricular junction.

- Failure of the membrane to reach the atrioventricular junction results in a low defect.

*To be read in conjunction with the following chapter.

Secundum ASD

While the foramen primum is closing a second hole appears in the membrane (foramen ovale). By the end of the fifth week another membrane forms to the right of the septum primum which forms a valve at the foramen ovale. This valve usually closes soon after birth by fusion of the primum and secundum septa.

- Failure of closure results in a secundum ASD.

Ventriculoseptal defects (VSD)

Division of the ventricle starts with the development of a central muscular ridge at the caudal end of the heart. This ridge grows towards the atrioventricular junction by proliferation of myoblasts. There is also growth of a thin membrane from the AV junction towards the muscular ridge. The septum is usually complete by the end of the seventh week.

- VSDs result from incomplete fusion of the membranous and muscular portion of the septum. Muscular portion VSDs are holes in the muscular septum.

Pulmonary/aortic stenosis

The pulmonary and aortic valves each derive from three swellings at the openings of the respective great vessels. The swellings develop into three thin walled cusps.

- Fusion of the cusps results in an opening which is too small to cope with the amount of blood that needs to go through the valve.

Tetralogy of Fallot (TOF)

- This malformation is a combination of a membranous VSD and pulmonary stenosis. These abnormalities result in overriding of the aorta and right ventricular hypertrophy.

Truncus arteriosus

The aorta and the pulmonary trunk derive from a single tube which is divided by the spiral aortico-pulmonary septum.

- Failure of formation results in persistent truncus arteriosus, i.e. a single outlet from the ventricles. This abnormality is always associated with a VSD.

Transposition of the great arteries

The embryological basis of this malformation is uncertain.

- A popular theory is that the aortico-pulmonary septum does not take a spiral course resulting in incorrect attachment of the vessels to the ventricles.

Patent ductus arteriosus

The ductus arteriosus is essential for normal fetal circulation. It joins the aorta to the pulmonary trunk resulting in blood bypassing the lungs when they do not require a huge blood supply.

- It usually closes soon after birth and failure to do so in term infants is pathological.

Coarctation of the aorta

The embryological basis is uncertain. There are three main views.

1 Muscle tissue from the ductus arteriosus is incorporated into the aorta. When the duct closes at birth the muscle contracts, forming a coarctation.
2 There may be abnormal involution of the left dorsal aorta which becomes incorporated into the aorta with the left subclavian artery.
3 Little blood flow through this region occurs during normal prenatal life. After birth the blood flow increases causing the diameter of the aorta to increase. If it does not enlarge then a coarctation occurs.

Many other malformations of the heart are possible, often as combinations of the above described anomalies.

Genetics

An increasing number of conditions are identified by chromosome DNA markers using fluorescence in situ hybridization (FISH). A good example is congenital heart disease associated with chromosome 22:

1 CATCH 22 = Cardiac defect, Abnormal facial appearance, Thymic dysplasia, Cleft palate, Hypocalcaemia from parathyroid dysplasia. This characterizes both Di George and velocardiofacial syndrome, which have the same deletion, at q11.2.
2 Isolated conotruncal cardiac defects (interrupted aortic arch, truncus arteriosus, tetralogy of Fallot). About 30% show a similar microdeletion to CATCH 22.

Others identified using FISH technology include Williams syndrome (infantile hypercalcaemia, supravalvular aortic stenosis, characteristic facies, learning disorder) which shows a deletion of the elastin gene at 7q11.23.

Age at presentation of cardiac abnormalities:

	Acyanotic	*Cyanotic*
Early		
First week	Hypoplastic left heart	Transposition of great arteries
	Patent ductus arteriosus in premature	Persistent fetal circulation
		Truncus arteriosus
	Coarctation	Atresia/stenosis pulmonary or tricuspid valves
	Myocarditis	
	Complete heart block	Ebstein's tricuspid valve anomaly
		Total anomalous pulmonary venous connection (TAPVC) infradiaphragmatic, in which flow is obstructed
Weeks/months		
	Volume overload L→R shunt e.g. ventriculoseptal defect, single ventricle	Fallot's tetralogy
		Tricuspid atresia
		Ebstein's
	TAPVC non obstructed – supracardiac or cardiac	TAPVC
	Pressure overload pulmonary hypertension pulmonary stenosis	
	Myocarditis	
	Arrhythmias: paroxysmal tachycardia	
Late	Pressure overload including systemic hypertension	Pulmonary hypertension as part of Eisenmenger's syndrome
	Bacterial endocarditis	
	Myocarditis	

Surgical advances

Occluder devices

- Coils for patent ductus arteriosus <4 mm, suitable for even very low birth weight infants.
- Clamshells (or 'double umbrellas') for atrial septal defects and some ventriculoseptal defects.
- Double umbrellas/buttons for moderate PDAs. Expensive device (£1500) compared with a coil (£50), and sheath too big to allow use in prematures.
- Coils to occlude arteriovenous malformations causing heart failure.

Balloon dilatation for

- Hot wire with radio frequency diathermy to cardiac catheter lodged against an atretic pulmonary or aortic valve, followed by balloon dilatation.

- Coarctation at site of ductal narrowing, not with a natural coarctation as this may lead to aneurysm formation.
- Aortic stenosis. In the neonate this reduces the need for early surgery which will be required later anyway to insert a replacement valve.

Stents for peripheral pulmonary artery stenoses

Other procedures

- Atrial septal defect: closure now done if shunt is >1.5:1.
- Coarctation repair: end to end preferred, or a long oblique incision to form a subclavian flap is also commonly done.
- Aortic stenosis: Ross procedure, using own pulmonary valve, is popular.
- Hypoplastic left heart: Norwood procedure still has a high mortality.
- Tetralogy of Fallot: primary correction sooner, now in early infancy, with 90% survival.
- Single ventricle/tricuspid atresia variants: 2-stage procedure
  (i) bidirectional Glenn (ii) modified Fontan with a conduit from inferior vena cava to pulmonary artery (total caval pulmonary connection) to reduce arrhythmias.

Therapeutic controversy

Digoxin in the neonate with Wolff–Parkinson–White not as satisfactory as flecainide (class I, lignocaine like) or sotalol (class II, a β-blocker, and class III activity).

Kawasaki disease

Aetiology

Superantigen reaction to staphylococcal infection.

Epidemiology, the UK picture

Incidence 4.1 per 100 000 children, 80% under 5 years old, 25% with coronary artery involvement, mortality 4%. Late heart disease is as yet an unquantified risk in those who appear to have made a complete recovery.

Pathogenesis

Inflammatory response associated with a vasculitis, particularly affecting small blood vessels, especially the coronaries, to form aneurysms.

Clinical

Classically, five features (atypically three or more) of the following are needed for diagnosis:

1   Temperature for 5 or more days.
2   Rash, erythematous, macular or multiforme.
3   Oedema of hands and feet, peeling of the skin of fingertips.
4   Conjunctivitis, bilateral.
5   Lips dry, cracked, peeling, erythematous; strawberry tongue; pharyngeal erythema.
6   Cervical lymphadenopathy, non-suppurative.

   Additional features:

   i   Cardiac complications 30%, mainly develop in first 12–28 days; thrombosis and aneurysms of the coronary vessels, myocarditis, arrhythmias, hypertension.
   ii Vasculitis: peripheral gangrene, thromboses of brain/heart.
   iii Arthritis 20%, diarrhoea 10%, aseptic meningitis 10%, also uveitis, pneumonia, hydrops of gallbladder, ileus, hepatosplenomegaly.

Investigations

Raised WBC, platelets ($>10^6$ per 10^9/l in severe vasculitis), ESR (>100 mm/hour); pyuria, proteinuria. ECG, chest X-ray, echocardiography of the coronary arteries.
Check ASOT, DNA binding, rheumatoid factor – should be negative.

Differential diagnosis

Post streptococcal, staphylococcal, enterovirus, adenovirus, measles, parvovirus, leptospirosis, infectious mononucleosis, drug reaction, Stevens-Johnson syndrome, juvenile rheumatoid arthritis.

Management

1   Aspirin 80–100 mg/kg/day for the first 14 days of illness, then 3–5 mg/kg to inhibit platelet aggregation for 8 weeks; never been shown to prevent coronary artery aneurysms.
2   Intravenous gammaglobulin (IVGG) 2 g/kg single infusion (superior to 0.4 g/kg/day for 4 days) in the first 10 days may prevent coronary artery aneurysms.
3   Follow up for >1 year looking for cardiac complications, continuing aspirin as long as vascular changes are present. Half of aneurysms regress spontaneously within 18 months.

Prognosis

Mortality 4% from coronary insufficiency in the first 3 months, commoner in boys than girls and those under a year. Death may be sudden and unexpected.
Recurrence is rare.

•   Rapid diagnosis of Kawasaki by exclusion is essential to reduce morbidity and mortality, and must be considered in any child with a febrile illness lasting 4–5 days. Only 60% in a UK series (Dillon *et al.* 1993) received both aspirin and IVGG, and less than a third were given IVGG within the first 10 days of illness.

Reference

Dillon R, Newton L, Rudd P T, Hall S M (1993) Management of Kawasaki disease. *Archives of Disease in Childhood*, **69**, 631–8.

Lyme disease

This spirochaetal infection (*Borrelia burgsdorferi*) is spread by a tick whose reservoir in the UK is mainly small mammals, and deer.

After an incubation period of 3–32 days a herald lesion appears: papule with influenza like symptoms, followed by erythema chronicum migrans for 3–4 weeks.

Weeks or months later: meningitis, myocarditis, arthritis. Treat with i.v. cefotaxime 75 mg/kg for 14–21 days.

Myocarditis is characterized by signs of congestive cardiac failure, severe tachycardia (occasionally other arrhythmias, e.g. heart block, paroxysmal tachycardia), quiet precordium and gallop rhythm. Cardiomegaly and pulmonary oedema on chest X-ray. ECG shows low voltage QRS (<5 mm in limb leads), inverted T waves, occasional Q waves in V_{5-6}, prolongation of QT. Echo shows dilatation, poor contraction and ejection fraction, +/- pericardial effusion.

Management

General principles of treatment of dilated congestive cardiac failure: digoxin, avoiding too rapid digitalization as myocardium may be overly sensitive. Diuretics reduce the fluid load.

Reduction in vasomotor tone: angiotensin-converting enzyme (ACE) inhibitors may be helpful. β-blockers used in chronic cases.

Transplant is the final option.

Controversy in myocarditis

In chronic viral and idiopathic dilated cardiomyopathy no comparative trials of immunosuppression or gamma globulin have been done, but are often used. (NB: The aetiology of cardiomyopathies in children is more varied than in adults. Exclude hypertrophy due to aortic stenosis, hypertension, hypothyroidism, lipodystrophy, Noonan's syndrome, Friedreich's disease).

Investigation of unexplained ventricular hypertrophy also includes metabolic (e.g. storage disorders, carnitine deficiency), familial (idiopathic hypertrophic, dystrophies), and genetic (e.g. mitochondrial cytopathies) studies.

Investigations: fasting blood glucose, lymphocytes for vacuolation, carnitine, lactate, pyruvate, amino acids, and urine for amino acids, organic acids, glycosaminoglycans. WBC for enzymes in metabolic storage disorders, e.g. Gaucher's, GM_1 and GM_2 gangliosidosis.

Further reading

Burch M (1994) Hypertrophic cardiomyopathy. *Archives of Diseases of Childhood*, **71**, 488–489

ABC OF RESUSCITATION OF INFANTS AND CHILDREN

Most children present with hypoxia from respiratory failure or in hypovolaemic shock, in contradistinction from adults with cardiac arrest.

1   Place on a firm surface. Summon help.
2   Look for chest movement, listen for breath sounds (cheek close to victim's mouth), feel expired air on your cheek.
3   *Breathing?* Yes → recovery position.

No → Airway

   i   Carefully sweep mouth cavity with swab round finger or suction to remove vomit; there is a danger of pushing a foreign body (FB) further down into the airway if FB is not considered.
   ii   'Tilt head backwards, and chin lift' to establish airway. This lifts the tongue off the posterior pharyngeal wall. NB: overextension will kink the soft trachea, excessive pressure under the jaw to the soft tissues of the mouth will force the tongue into the airway.
   iii   If still not breathing consider obstruction by:

      a. Epiglottitis.
      b. Foreign body (FB) management:
         Infants: turn upside down and deliver 4 firm blows to the back.
         Children: abdominal compression by upward thrust of fist in the midline above the umbilicus (Heimlich manoeuvre) may move a FB upwards enough to grasp in older children.

Breathing

If still not breathing start mouth to mouth (or mouth and nose), gently breathing into the child until the chest wall rises adequately. Low pressure gives adequate volume avoiding gastric distension.

    Best is endotracheal intubation + ventilate by hand, next is oral airway + IPPV via a tight fitting mask with oxygen. Give 4 breaths initially.

    Rate: Infant 24/minute, child 20/minute.

    Use an uncuffed tube under 8 years old to avoid pressure necrosis to the trachea.

4   Circulation

Feel for the brachial pulse, alternatively use the carotid or femoral. If inadequate rate or volume, start chest compression. The heart lies under the lower sternum. Surface marking in a child is 2 finger breadths below the line joining the nipples.

Infant: apply pressure with both thumbs on the sternum, fingers encircling the chest.

Toddler: 2 fingers on the sternum, the other hand under the back (suitable for infants too). If a large toddler, use the heel of one hand, compressing 1.5–2.5 cm.

Child: heel of 2 hands, adult style, compressing 2.5–3.5 cm.

  i   Smooth compression, not too rapid, enough to produce a pulse.
  ii Rate 100–120/minute.
  iii Release pressure between strokes to allow the sternum to return to its normal position, and time for the ventricles to fill.

Count aloud 1 + 2 + 3 + 4 + 5, then breathe into a small child; 15 compressions to 2 breaths into an older child, or if without an assistant.

5   *Drugs* (Table 2.1)

Establish i.v., or more rapidly, intraosseous access during resuscitation.

Controversy: hyperosmolar alkali infusions in cardiopulmonary resuscitation may compromise the outcome by reducing coronary perfusion. If the colour remains poor after 5–10 minutes, or frankly cyanosed, sodium bicarbonate 8.4% 1–2 ml/kg and glucose 25% 1–2 ml/kg may be given at the discretion of the resuscitation team leader, preferably after obtaining bloods for pH, glucose, biochemistry, etc.

Further action is rarely required as children usually have healthy myocardia.

6   *ECG*

Cardiac drugs are given according to the ECG trace. If ECG monitoring is unavailable, it is assumed that asystole is present.

  i   Asystole: adrenaline is effective if instilled via the ET tube or may be given i.v. Avoid the intracardiac route.
  ii Bradycardia: atropine *first*, as it may be vagally mediated, then adrenaline/isoprenaline.
  iii Ventricular fibrillation/tachycardia: DC shock 1 joule/kg. Double and redouble dose if no response. Consider lignocaine, then bretylium, applying DC shock each time.
      If asystole follows, give adrenaline.

Table 2.1   Drugs useful in cardiorespiratory arrest

Drug	Dose (volume)	Indication
Adrenaline* 1:10 000	10 µg/kg (0.1 ml/kg)	Asystole, severe anaphylaxis
Atropine* (600 µg/ml)	<1 year 0.1 ml, 1–4 years 0.2 ml 5 years 0.3 ml, 12 years 0.6 ml	Atrial bradycardia/vagal stimulation
Ca gluconate* (10%)	1 ml/year, maximum 10 ml	Hyperkalaemia Verapamil antidote
Dobutamine	2.5–10 µg/kg/min+	Low cardiac output
Dopamine*	2–4 µg/kg/min**	Renal shut down: reduced perfusion
	10–20 µg/kg/min	Cardiogenic shock
Lignocaine 1%	0.5–1 mg/kg (0.05–0.1 ml/kg) 20–50 µg/kg/min	Ventricular tachyarrhythmia
Mannitol 20%	2.5–5 ml/kg	Cerebral oedema
Sodium bicarbonate 8.4%	1–5 mmol/kg (1–5 ml/kg)	Severe acidosis

*Inactivated if mixed with sodium bicarbonate
+Add 2 ml/kg from 250 mg in 20 ml ampoule to 50 ml 5% dextrose. Rate 0.3–1.2 ml/h
**Add 0.5 ml/kg from 200 mg in 5 ml ampoule to 50 ms 5% dextrose. Rate 0.3–0.6 ml/h

6   Failure of circulation due to shock

If dehydration or pre-existing hypovolaemia is the likely cause of the arrest give albumin/haemaccel/dextrose saline by syringe, 20 ml/kg, as rapidly as possible to a total of 60 ml in the first hour. Follow up with dobutamine or dopamine infusion.

7   Cerebral oedema, renal failure, consumption coagulopathy require to be anticipated (see relevant sections).

Further reading

Carcillo J A, Davis A L, Zaritsky A (1991) Role of early fluid resuscitation in pediatric septic shock. *Journal of the American Medical Association*, **286**, 1242–1245
Ryder I G, Munro H M, Doull I J M Intraosseous infusion for resuscitation. *Archives of Disease in Childhood*, **66**, 1442–1443

HYPOTENSION

Causes are hypovolaemia, cardiogenic shock, or peripheral pooling (Table 2.2). All can lead to coma.

Table 2.2   Important causes of shock

Hypovolaemia	Cardiogenic	Peripheral pooling
Haemorrhage	Tension pneumothorax	Septic shock
Gastroenteritis	Pericardial effusion	Anaphylaxis
Diabetes mellitus and insipidus	Arrhythmias	Drugs: e.g. barbiturate
Hypoadrenalism	Congenital heart disease	Toxic shock syndrome
	Cardiomyopathy	

Assessment

1 The history

Vital to determining the cause.

Examples: trauma; access to drugs; infection – contacts or symptoms; sting or medication; increased or reduced voiding of urine; tampon use in an adolescent girl; known heart disease, diabetes, sickle cell, allergies.

2 Clinical

i Smell: ketones, e.g. diabetes, starvation, hypoglycaemia.
ii Skin: cyanosis, pallor, dehydration, rashes, trauma. *Capillary refill time >2 seconds.*
iii Neurology: coma, focal signs, meningism, fundi for raised intracranial pressure.
iv Trunk:

- Ventilatory effort, added breath sounds.
- Cardiac arrhythmia or failure, a murmur indicating heart disease.
- Abdominal distension in necrotizing enterocolitis, surgical or infective problem.
  Organomegaly, e.g. splenic sequestration.
  Mass, e.g. haematoma.
- Genitalia pigmented or ambiguous in congenital adrenal hyperplasia.

Investigations

1 Blood gases to establish severity of acidosis (usually from hypoperfusion) and hypoventilation.
2 Blood count, blood cultures, coagulation screen.
   WBC count may be raised in infection or stress, or low if overwhelming infection; consumption coagulopathy occurs in septic shock and hypovolaemic shock.
3 Serum electrolytes and urea, liver function and blood glucose. May identify major electrolyte deficits/excess and organ failure (e.g. renal, or liver in Reye's syndrome).
4 Blood and urine for drug screen, organic and amino acids.
5 Cultures from septic sites, suprapubic urine aspiration, stool, and vagina if toxic shock syndrome is suspected in an adolescent. A lumbar puncture may be delayed if too sick, or raised intracranial pressure likely, as CSF antibodies to common microorganisms can be identified later.
6 Chest X-ray is likely to show pulmonary plethora in cardiogenic shock and peripheral pooling. Widespread or local consolidation in pneumonia. Sometimes little to see in the early stages, especially in staphylococcal pneumonia.
   Heart shape and size may be diagnostic.
7 ECG abnormalities of rhythm, e.g. supraventricular tachycardia, or strain patterns indicative as in endocardial fibroelastosis.

Management

Monitoring: insert a urinary catheter and consider central venous pressure monitoring. Continuous ECG, frequent BP measurement, core-periphery temperature difference ($>3°C$ is significant).

1   Fluids

   i   Blood/plasma expander 20 ml/kg over 20 minutes.
   ii   In septic shock, give plasma quickly, followed by dextrose-saline to a total of 60 ml in the first hour, and 120 ml/kg within the first 6 h.
   iii Dopamine can be added in hypovolaemic states.

2   Pressor agent, e.g. dobutamine for cardiogenic shock.
3   Diuretic for systemic or pulmonary oedema.
4   Steroids in large dose if:

   i   Septic or toxic shock is likely.
   ii   Response to resuscitation is incomplete: adrenal shock is possible, e.g. Waterhouse–Friderichsen syndrome.
   iii Anaphylaxis. First give an antihistamine and adrenaline subcutaneously or i.v.

5   Sodium bicarbonate: may give 1–2 ml/kg or base excess $\times$ 0.3 $\times$ body weight.
6   Antibiotics if indicated: penicillin and gentamicin or ampicillin and chloramphenicol or ceftazidime and flucloxacillin are standard broad spectrum combinations. Metronidazole may be added if an anaerobic infection is suspected, e.g. an immunocompromised child.

Further reading

Fleisher G R, Ludwig S (1988) *Textbook of Pediatric Emergency Medicine* 2nd edn. Baltimore, MD: Williams & Wilkins
Rogers M C (1987) *Textbook of Pediatric Intensive Care* Baltimore, MD: Williams & Wilkins
Selbst S M, Torrey S B (1988) *Pediatric Emergency Medicine for the House Officer* Baltimore, MD:Williams & Wilkins, useful algorithms

Chapter 3

Cardiovascular problems

DEVELOPMENT OF THE HEART AND CONGENITAL HEART DISEASE

The heart begins in the third week of fetal life as a tube and within 4 weeks is a complex 4-chambered and valved organ.

Dextrocardia occurs if the tube bends to the left instead of the right. Defects are common if it is isolated, and uncommon with situs inversus when all the viscera are transposed.

Teratogenic influence

Vulnerable period 15–60 days fetal age.

Causes

Mainly multifactorial.

Others

1   Hereditary, e.g. AD as in Marfan's and Noonan's syndromes, some atrial septal defects, and hypertrophic obstructive cardiomyopathy.
2   Chromosomal, e.g. Down's syndrome, trisomy 13, 18, Turner's syndrome.
3   Maternal disease:

   i Diabetes

      a. Persistent: transposition of the great arteries (TGA), ventricular septal defect (VSD), single ventricle, hypoplastic left heart.
      b. Transient hypertrophic cardiomyopathy resolves by 6 months.

   ii Rubella: patent ductus arteriosus (PDA), pulmonary valve stenosis, branch and central pulmonary artery stenosis, coarctation of the aorta.
   iii Alcohol: VSD, ASD.
         Drugs: lithium and Ebstein anomaly; phenytoin and VSD or ASD.
   iv Phenylketonuria: tetralogy of Fallot, VSD, coarctation of aorta.
   v Systemic lupus erythematosus: complete heart block by Ro antibody.

4   Monozygotic twins.

CONGENITAL HEART DISEASE (CHD)

With renal anomalies, the commonest of persistent congenital abnormalities.

Natural history

25% would die in the neonatal period, 60% in infancy, and only 15% survive to adolescence. Altered by surgical repair and palliation.

Acquired disease is less common in developed countries where rheumatic heart disease and symptomatic infections are rare.

Incidence of congenital heart abnormalities

5–7 per 1000 live births.
Commonest nine overall in the UK (80% of all cases):
Ventriculoseptal defect (VSD) 30%.
2nd equal at 8% each: persistent patent ductus arteriosus (PDA), pulmonary stenosis (PS), atrioseptal defect (ASD).
5th equal: tetralogy of Fallot (TF), coarctation of aorta, aortic stenosis 6% each.
8th equal: transposition of great vessels (TGA), atrioventricular (AV) defect 4% each.
Commonest six in the first year
VSD (15%), TGA (10%), TF (9%), coarctation (8%), hypoplastic left heart (7%), PDA (6%).

Genetic risk and antenatal detection

1   General advice

Other than in Mendelian inherited conditions, the recurrence risk is small, bearing in mind the incidence of a fetal abnormality in any pregnancy is 3%.

 i Siblings 1–3%, and about 10% for left heart obstructive lesions like coarctation and hypoplastic left heart.
 ii Offspring of an affected parent 2–4%, may be higher for some individual lesions.

2   Antenatal diagnosis by US

Optimal US examination, including a four chamber view, e.g. to detect hypoplastic left heart defects, is at 18–24 weeks' gestation, with the option of also performing chromosome analysis if appropriate. For example, detection of a complete atrioventricular septal defect may indicate a trisomy 21 which the mother may prefer terminated. If a hypoplastic left heart, termination is likely to be offered as the treatment option has a very high mortality.

Other situations benefiting from US examination:

i   High risk families with existing CHD in a first degree relative.
ii Diabetic mothers, and those taking possibly teratogenic drugs.
iii Other fetal abnormalities: arrhythmias, ascites, non-cardiac abnormalities seen on US.
iv Increasingly as part of the routine US examination in all pregnancies.

Further reading

Allen L D (1989) Diagnosis of fetal cardiac abnormalities. *Archives of Disease in Childhood*, **64**, 964–968
Allan L D, Cook D, Sullivan I, Sharland G K (1991) Hypoplastic left heart syndrome: effects of fetal echocardiography on birth prevalence. *Lancet*, i, 959–961
Lin A E, Garver K L (1988) Genetic counseling for congenital heart defects. *Journal of Pediatrics*, **113**, 1105–1109

Some associated syndromes

(Useful 'handles' to identify underlying heart disease>)

1   Asymmetric crying face (septal defects +/– renal, vertebral anomalies, anal atresia).
2   Ellis–van Crefeld syndrome AR: atrioseptal defect, short limbed dwarf, polydactyly, small nails.
3   Kartagener syndrome AR: situs invertus (50%), bronchiectasis, sinusitis, sterility in males due to abnormal dien arms in cilia structure.
4   Noonan syndrome: 1 in 2500; 50% have pulmonary stenosis, atrioseptal defect, or septal hypertrophy.
5   Williams syndrome: supravalvular aortic stenosis, 'elfin face', hypercalcaemia.
6   Associations: VACTERL association: expansion of VATER to include cardiac (VSD, ASD, PDA, Fallot's tetralogy) and limb defects. Incidence 1 in 6000. CHARGE association.

EVALUATION OF HEART DISEASE

1   Age at presentation is a useful guide to the underlying lesion (Table 3.1).

Table 3.1   Age at presentation (a rough guide)

Hours or days	Atresia of pulmonary or aortic valve
Days to week	Hypoplastic left heart, complex defect, e.g. TGA, Fallot's tetralogy
One to 3 months	Large left to right shunt, e.g. VSD, PDA
Three months to one year	Fallot's tetralogy, endocardial fibroelastosis, paroxysmal atrial tachycardia, Kawasaki disease
Over one year	Eisenmenger syndrome, systemic hypertension, bacterial endocarditis

2   Symptoms of cardiac decompensation

   i   Dyspnoea and slow to complete feeds. In infancy, the effort required is equivalent to an exercise test of cardiorespiratory reserve.

   ii   Cyanosis.

   iii   Dry cough and wheeze due to pulmonary oedema.

   iv   Pallor/shock due to low systemic BP. Sweating, and crying persistently.

   v   Excessive, rapid weight gain (>30 g/day) from fluid retention.

3   Precipitating factors

   i   Infection, especially respiratory ⎱ Either can cause
   ii   Anaemia   ⎰ acute cardiac failure.

4   Specific symptoms:
Squatting in tetralogy of Fallot.
Chest pain in aberrant coronary arteries, plus syncope in aortic valve stenosis.
Lassitude, fever, anaemia, and purpura in bacterial endocarditis.

5   Pregnancy: rubella, alcohol, drugs, maternal diabetes.

6   Family history: see genetic aspects.

Examination

1   Observation

   i   Abnormal facies/malformations in 10% of infants with CHD.

   ii   Mucous membranes for anaemia, cyanosis, digits (fingers and toes) for clubbing.

Cyanosis

Present in the following situations:

   i   Newborn with high haematocrit, with otherwise normal oxygen content, if >5 g/dl Hb desaturated.

   ii   If >1.5 g/dl reduced Hb, providing the child is not anaemic, when pallor masks the cyanosis.

   iii   Central: the tongue is most reliable, as the gums may be darkly pigmented in Asians and Blacks.

   iv   Peripheral: hands and feet blue.
Normal in neonates.
Common finding in pyrexial illness as core temperature rises.
Shock.

   v   Traumatic: head blue and purpuric from neck compression by umbilical cord/force.

   vi   Differential

      a.   Coarctation of the aorta with patent ductus → pink upper trunk, cyanosed below.

      b.   Transposition of the great arteries with pulmonary hypertension → patent ductus arteriosus → cyanosed upper trunk, pink below.

Causes of central cyanosis

1 Central depression: drugs, immaturity, trauma, asphyxia.
2 Seizures.
3 Respiratory disease.

   i V/Q imbalance, e.g. pneumonia, pneumothorax, atelectasis.
   ii Airway obstruction (choanal atresia, laryngeal/tracheal obstruction).

4 Shock: septicaemia, hypoglycaemia, adrenal crisis.
5 Polycythaemia in the newborn.
6 Cardiac disease.
7 Methaemoglobinaemia.

Assessment

1 History, chest X-ray, ECG, right radial (preductal) artery blood gas.
2 *Hyperoxia test*, breathing 100% oxygen for 10 minutes. Positive for CHD = arterial PaO_2 of less than 20 kPa, in the absence of severe lung disease, or vigorous crying in a normal infant leading to intrapulmonary shunting. Rarely, an infant with significant mixing of systemic and pulmonary blood will appear pink, during the test, due to massive pulmonary blood flow.

Respiration and pulse

A respiration:pulse rate ratio of less than 3:1 is suggestive of a respiratory cause:

	Respiration/minute	Pulse/minute
Infant/toddler:	30 +/– 10	100 +/– 20
Child:	25 +/– 10	90 +/– 10

   i Palpate all 4 limb pulses and carotids.

- Delay or absence of femorals in coarctation may be difficult to evaluate in the infant.
- In a shocked neonate, absent left radial or carotid pulse points to an interrupted aortic arch.
- Carotid thrill is found in left ventricular outlet obstruction, e.g. aortic stenosis.

   ii Weak pulse = poor peripheral circulation: e.g. septic shock, dehydration, cardiac:

     a. In the neonate, aortic stenosis, hypoplastic left heart, coarctation with endocardial fibroelastosis, infective cardiomyopathy.
     b. At older ages, cardiac failure from many causes.

   iii Full, 'bounding' pulses: temperature, thyrotoxicosis, arteriovenous fistula, cardiac mixing with rapid pressure 'run off', e.g. patent ductus arteriosus, truncus arteriosus, aortopulmonary window.

3   Auscultation in infants and toddlers, before undressing which is often resented, and can result in crying. Lift vest/shirt or even listen through it!

4   Inspection. Once undressed look for:

i   Neck pulsations: increased in PDA, aortic incompetence, and thyrotoxicosis.

ii Venous engorgement as a sign of cardiac failure: in <2 year olds it is more reliable to assess liver size.

iii Precordial bulge = right ventricular hypertrophy. Thoracotomy and sterniotomy scars are indicative of palliative/reparative surgery to the heart and/or lungs.

iv Oedema over sacrum/around the eyes in recumbent infants.

5   Palpation

i   Precordium. Always check for dextrocardia.

a. Apex beat. Impulse ++ from increased left ventricle stroke volume, e.g. VSD, and prolonged in outlet obstruction, e.g. aortic stenosis, coarctation. Left parasternal heave = right ventricular enlargement.

b. Thrills are systolic, caused by forcing blood through a small diameter hole, e.g. VSD or narrowed aortic or pulmonary valve.

c. Palpable pulmonary second sound in second left interspace = pulmonary hypertension.

ii Liver edge: normally 1–3 cm below the costal margin in nipple line. Enlargement in cardiac failure. Beware of apparent enlargement from the liver being pushed down by respiratory disease/lobar emphysema/subphrenic abscess.

6   Blood pressure
Take the blood pressure once you have gained the child's confidence. The cuff must cover most of the upper arm, with the bladder completely encircling the arm. In infants the Doppler method is commonly used, or the more traditional flush test which measures mean BP.
Normal range:

Age	Median BP	95th centile for systolic BP (mmHg)
Neonate	75	95
2–14 years	95	115

The BP is usually 20 mmHg higher in the legs, so reversal of normal suggests coarctation.
Diastolic may be indeterminate even in healthy children.

Hypertension

Hypertension = >95th centile. Population screening is not justified. Obesity is the commonest association, and requires diet and sodium restriction.

Risk factors: neonatal umbilical artery catheterization. A family history of renal polycystic disease or phaeochromocytoma.

Select renal disease, diabetes mellitus, neurofibromatosis, and familial hypertension for follow up.

Pathological causes:

  i In the first year renal vascular abnormalities (secondary to umbilical arterial thrombi, renal artery stenosis (RAS), renal vein thrombosis) and coarctation are the commonest causes.
 ii In early childhood mainly renal abnormality (90%):

    a. 80%: reflux nephropathy, chronic glomerulonephritis, haemolytic uraemic syndrome, obstructive uropathy, (neurogenic or structural).

    b. 10% renal vascular abnormalities (e.g. RAS in von Recklinghausen disease).

       Presentations: failure to thrive, headache, facial palsy.

       Investigate for a and b with US, DMSA, DTPA renal scans and/or micturating cystogram, peripheral and renal vein plasma renin, and angiography of the renal vein.

       Remaining 10%:

    1 Raised intracranial pressure.
    2 Tumours, e.g. neuroblastoma, phaeochromocytoma, Wilm's.
    3 Endocrine: congenital adrenal hyperplasia, Cushing syndrome, primary hyperaldosteronism.

       Characteristic clinical findings with imaging of tumours and urinary amines or steroid excretion.

iii Older children: obesity and essential hypertension are most likely, and unless secondary hypertension is suspected, examination, family history, normal urinalysis, sterile urine, normal serum electrolytes, bicarbonate and creatinine suffice.

Management of hypertension

1 Surgery for appropriate cases.
2 Mild, and essential hypertension: weight reduction, salt restriction, exercise.
3 Moderate to severe: first try a thiazide diuretic or frusemide, next a β-blocker, finally a vasodilator. Hyper-reninaemia secondary to renal hypertension responds well to the angiotensin converting enzyme (ACE) inhibitor captopril.
4 Hypertensive crisis: the vasodilator sodium nitroprusside, except in acute post infectious glomerulonephritis, when frusemide alone is usually sufficient.

Drug doses

Captopril 0.5–2 mg/kg twice daily.
Chlorthiazide 10 mg/kg twice daily.
Frusemide 1–2 mg/kg two to three times daily.
Hydralazine 0.5 mg/kg three times daily (idiosyncratic hypotension is a danger, so always give a test dose).
Propranolol 0.5–1 mg/kg three times daily, up to 2 mg/kg/dose.
Sodium nitroprusside 0.5–1 μg/kg/minute.

Further reading

Report of the Second Task Force on Blood Pressure Control in Children (1987) *Pediatrics*, **79**, 1–25

AUSCULTATION

Order:

1   Heart sounds, concentrating on the second: if single = pathological

Normally the aortic valve closes before the pulmonary valve. The gap widens in inspiration, and its absence requires an explanation. If the younger child cannot regulate breathing, the first few beats on sitting up after lying down will bring out the presence of splitting.

- i   Single and loud in pulmonary hypertension when pulmonary artery pressure approaches systemic, as in a large VSD, where the systolic murmur may disappear as the pressures become equal, i.e. becoming an Eisenmenger's syndrome. Only the quality of the heart sound indicates the severity of the condition.
- ii   Single and soft in aortic stenosis or hypoplastic left heart, and may even be so delayed as to give reversed splitting, i.e. wider in expiration.

Split, fixed and usually wide in ASD, though it may be narrow in infancy, only to be detected in later childhood as the heart rate falls.

Split widely, varying with respiration, with soft second sound in isolated pulmonary stenosis or Fallot's tetralogy (may sound single).

First heart sound: loud in mitral stenosis (rare).

2   Added sounds

Third heart sound during early ventricular filling, is low pitched (best heard with bell):

- i   Physiological and heard in 20% of normal hearts.
- ii   Pathological gallop due to a dilated, poorly contracting, or failing, left ventricle, as in aortic stenosis, or myocarditis.

Ejection click

- i   High frequency, heard in early systole = stenosis with post-stenotic dilatation of aorta or pulmonary artery. Click is absent if the valve is thickened or severely dysplastic.

   Diagnostic confusion occurs when 'aortic clicks' are heard due to truncus arteriosus, dilatation of the aortic root in pulmonary atresia or Fallot's tetralogy, but the infant is more usually cyanosed in these states.

Site aids identification. Pulmonary valve abnormalities in the pulmonary area (left upper sternal border), aortic at the apex.

ii Mid systole = mitral valve prolapse.

3 Murmurs

Listen in systole, then diastole. A murmur may be physiological in systole but never in diastole (*cave* venous hums).

Systolic murmurs

In general, these are due to impeded flow, the intensity proportional to the pressure gradient. Low frequency murmurs are likely to produce a thrill as in VSD or aortic stenosis, but not with high pitched murmurs as in mitral regurgitation.

i Ejection 'diamond shaped' murmur = high pressure gradient due to obstruction or increased flow:

  a. *Narrow* semilunar valves in:

- aortic stenosis: apical murmur, associated with a carotid thrill, +/– apical click;
- pulmonary stenosis: second left interspace, single second sound or soft pulmonary component. If a pulmonary click is present, the earlier it occurs the more severe the stenosis.

  b. Normal valves with *increased flow*:

- ASD (fixed splitting of the second sound).
- VSD with high pulmonary pressure raising right ventricular pressure, and only the loud second sound is a warning of this potentially irreversible danger.

ii Pansystolic murmur = low pressure gradient, either through a shunt, or regurgitation through a valve:

  a. *Shunt*: site, radiation and intensity are of help in older infants.

- e.g. VSD, best heard at left sternal border, radiating to the apex and through to the lower back. Loudness is proportional to size, i.e. soft in a small VSD; may be shortened towards the end of systole if due to small muscular defects which close during the contraction.
- PDA, subclavicular, radiating through to the left scapula area. Found in infancy, in which pressures in the aorta and pulmonary artery are equal in diastole at which point no flow occurs across it.

  b. *Regurgitant*: incompetent mitral/tricuspid valve.

- Lower left sternal border (difficult to differentiate from VSD): tricuspid due to persistent pulmonary hypertension in the neonate or obstructed right ventricular outflow as in pulmonary atresia and Ebstein's anomaly.

- Blowing, apical, radiating to the axilla: mitral incompetence. Differentiate from mild mitral valve prolapse, found in up to 5% of normal children and Marfan's syndrome, with its loud mid-systolic click and late systolic murmur using the diaphragm, and not usually heard in infancy.

Diastolic murmurs are always pathological

i Early diastolic, soft and high pitched: incompetent semilunar aortic or pulmonary valve. Use the diaphragm down the left sternal edge, child sitting forward, holding breath in expiration.

   a. Common after valvotomy for aortic stenosis, valvotomy and repair of Fallot's tetralogy.
   b. To-and-fro murmur. A combination of ejection systolic with early diastolic murmur in the aortic area and lower left sternal edge is indicative of an abnormal and incompetent valve as in:

   - truncus arteriosus (often with an early systolic click), or
   - subvalvular aortic stenosis (no click).
   - Absent pulmonary valve is similar, heard in the pulmonary area.

ii Middle diastole, tends to be a low pitched rumble. Use the bell:

   a. Usually across normal valves with increased flow due to shunts. Its presence indicates that the ratio of flow through the shunt of pulmonary to systemic circulations is >2:1.
      Tricuspid: lower left sternal edge, increasing on inspiration in ASD, and anomalous pulmonary venous connection.
      Mitral: apical in PDA, VSD.
   b. Stenotic mitral valve in obstructive left heart conditions.

iii Late diastole/presystole: obstructed flow across a 'tight' mitral valve; a VSD's increased flow will accentuate it. Low pitched, rumbling, best heard with the bell.

Continuous murmurs

A pressure difference is present throughout the cardiac cycle.

i Patent ductus arteriosus in 90% (usually systolic alone in infancy).
ii Combinations of AS and AI, MI and AI, VSD and AI.
iii Collateral circulation, best heard over the back:

   a. Acyanotic: aortic in coarctation of the aorta, >5 years old.
   b. Cyanosed: bronchial collaterals in pulmonary atresia + VSD.

Venous hum, being continuous, may cause confusion, but it disappears on lying down, applying pressure over the neck veins, or in a Valsava manoeuvre.

Innocent murmurs

Characteristics are:

i Asymptomatic.
ii Heart sounds are normal.
iii The murmur is systolic, short ejection. Never diastolic.
iv Intensity: soft, grade 3/6 or less.
v Localized usually to the left of the sternum. No radiation through to the back.
vi Varies with posture.

Other innocent types heard in childhood

- Venous hum, see above.
- Vibratory: like the buzzing of a bee, becoming softer if sat up and the neck extended.
- Pulmonary systolic murmur (upper left chest → infraclavicular region) with normal splitting in inspiration. Differential is from mild pulmonary stenosis, where a widely split second sound is heard, with ECG and chest X-ray changes.

Investigations

Chest X-ray

Assess cardiac size, presence of pulmonary artery or right-sided aorta, and lung field vascularity. Classic shape, e.g. Fallot's 'coeur en sabot', is absent in 50%.
    Important features to be noted:

1 Cardiomegaly = cardiothoracic ratio of >0.50, due to: congestive cardiac failure, pericardial effusion, myocarditis, cardiomyopathy, complete heart block, Ebstein's malformation.
    Thymus shadow can confuse. The sail/wave signs help to differentiate. Rapid thymic involution in cyanosis/stress.
2 Absent pulmonary artery shadow in pulmonary stenosis/atresia, Fallot's tetralogy, TGA, truncus arteriosus, and tricuspid atresia.
3 A right-sided aortic arch is seen in Fallot's tetralogy (20%), pulmonary atresia with VSD. Less common are TGA and truncus arteriosus.
4 Notched ribs, due to collaterals in coarctation of the aorta, are seen from 5 years old.
5 Lung fields and pulmonary blood flow (PBF).

- Increased vascularity (PBF) in left to right shunts.

    i Acyanotic: PDA, VSD, ASD, atrioventricular canal.
    ii Cyanotic: TGA, truncus arteriosus, single ventricle.

- Venous congestion (hazy lung fields) if back pressure occurs, e.g. heart failure from coarctation, aortic stenosis, hypoplastic left heart, total anomalous pulmonary venous connection (TAPVC).
- Decreased vascularity (PBF).

    i Acyanotic: Pulmonary stenosis. In pulmonary hypertension a 'pruned' appearance with loss of vascular markings towards the periphery of the lung.

ii   Cyanotic: Fallot's tetralogy, atresia of pulmonary/tricuspid valve, Ebstein's malformation.

Electrocardiogram (Figure 3.1 and Table 3.2)

Normal findings:

QRS axis moves anticlockwise with age.

Table 3.2   Selected ECG changes

Type	Cause
1 Ventricular hypertrophy: the R wave changes	
i *Right ventricular hypertrophy* $V_4R > 15$ mm if < 3 months old $V_4R > 10$ mm if > 3 months old	1 Acyanotic: pulmonary stenosis 2 Cyanotic: Fallot's TGA, pulmonary hypertension
ii *Left ventricular hypertrophy* V6 > 20 mm if < 3 months old V6 > 25 mm if > 3 months old	Acyanotic: shunts, left heart obstruction and/or valve incompetence, cardiomyopathy, endocardial fibroelastosis
iii *Biventricular hypertrophy* Sum of R+S waves > 70 mm	VSD
2 QRS negative in 1, aVF, + RBBB QRS negative in 1, aVF, no RBBB	Atrioventricular defect Tricuspid atresia
3 RBBB of rsR in V_1, prolonged PR RBBB +/– complete heart block	ASD secundum After surgery for Fallot's, VSD
4 Short PR, broad QRS with δ wave	Wolff Parkinson White syndrome

Echocardiography

Cross-sectional echocardiography shows anatomical detail, pericardial effusions, vegetations. Doppler echocardiography gives information on flow rates and patterns, and gradients of pressure across valves.

Cardiac catheterization

Indications now few, as information is more safely obtained by echocardiography. One such is pulmonary artery pressure in pulmonary hypertension, as operability depends on the severity of pulmonary vascular resistance. However, the velocity of a regurgitant jet from the pulmonary valve, or flow across a PDA, can be measured by Doppler, so catheterization may be unnecessary.

Normal catheterization data

1   Oxygen saturation (%)   right heart   75 +/– 5
                            left heart   97 +/– 2

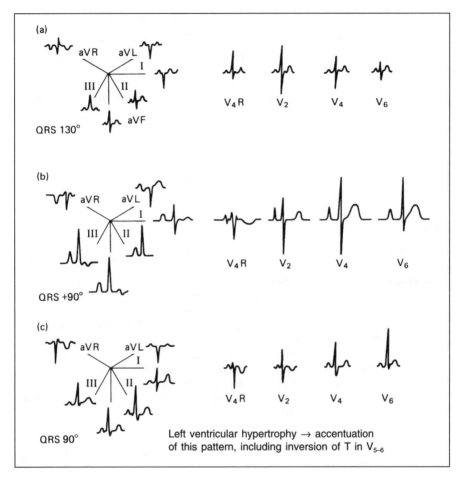

Figure 3.1
a. Newborn normal ECG, with positive QRS complexes in right chest leads, aVR, III and
V_4R. At older ages right ventricular hypertrophy has a similar or more accentuated pattern.
b. By contrast, a neonate with pulmonary atresia and intact ventricular septum showing
severely reduced right ventricular activity for age, and tall P waves
c. A child up to 8 years old. Positive complexes in II, aVF, III, and inverted T waves from
V_4R to V_3

2   Pressure in mmHg:

right atrium	3–7
left atrium	10–13
right ventricle	25/0
left ventricle	90–120/0
pulmonary artery	25/10
aorta	90–120/50–80
pulmonary arterial wedge	10–13

COMMON PRESENTATIONS OF CHD IN THE NEWBORN AND INFANT, BASIC MECHANISMS AND DIFFERENTIATION FROM NON-CARDIAC CAUSES

Presentation is usually with cyanosis, and/or heart failure, and occasionally as an arrhythmia.

Cyanosis

Mechanism: abnormal connection of great vessels, obstruction to flow, or mixing of systemic and pulmonary circulation.

Examples in the newborn

1   Inadequate mixing. Aorta arising from the right ventricle as in transposition of the great arteries (TGA).
2   Obstructive +/– intracardiac defect:
   i   Pulmonary valve atresia/critical stenosis +/– ventriculoseptal defect (VSD) or patent ductus arteriosus (PDA).
   ii Pulmonary artery vasoconstriction (dynamic): persistent fetal circulation through a PDA.
   iii Small ventricles: hypoplastic left heart, Ebstein's malformation in which the tricuspid valve is displaced into the right ventricle.
3   Mixing of systemic and pulmonary venous blood as in total anomalous pulmonary venous connection (TAPVC) with obstruction to venous return, and in truncus arteriosus.

Cyanosis, presenting in infancy, caused by mixing of systemic and pulmonary circulations

   i   Fallot's tetralogy, tricuspid atresia, Ebstein's, TAPVC, complete atrioventricular defect, or truncus arteriosus.
   ii Acyanotic progressing to cyanotic heart disease:

   Large VSD or ASD with pulmonary hypertension = Eisenmenger syndrome, following the reversal of a L → R shunt in VSD, transposition of the great arteries, and Down's syndrome with VSD or atrioventricular defect. Fortunately rare before 2 years in a simple VSD.

Heart failure

Presentation

Tachypnoea, tachycardia, excessive weight gain, wheeze.
   Pathophysiology due to at least one of the following mechanisms:

1   Obstruction (pressure overload): hypoplastic left heart, coarctation of the aorta, aortic stenosis.
2   Hyperdynamic (volume overload) circulation: PDA, truncus arteriosus.

Large arteriovenous fistula in the cranium or liver are rare but warrant auscultation of these organs.
3 Pump failure (myocarditis) is unusual: viral, ischaemia, metabolic.
4 Incomplete diastolic filling (constrictive pericarditis, pericardial effusion, chronic tachycardias) is rare.

VSD and PDA, the common causes after 3–4 weeks old, are usually asymptomatic before the fall in pulmonary vascular resistance.

Absence of a heart murmur does not exclude heart disease and is not uncommon in TGA, TAPVC, hypoplastic left heart, and coarctation of the aorta.

Acyanotic heart disease may present as cyanotic, secondary to cardiac failure and respiratory difficulty.

Differential diagnosis

Cyanotic congenital heart disease (CHD) has to be differentiated from:

- Respiratory problems.
- Persistent pulmonary hypertension.
- Myocardial malfunction.
- Arrhythmias.

Rarely, chocolate coloured blood with the slate blue cyanosis of methaemoglobinaemia is found.

1 Respiratory disorder

If cyanotic CHD is suspected many do a hyperoxia/nitrogen wash out test, obtaining blood gases in air and after 10 minutes in 100% oxygen. The PaO_2 should rise to >20 kPa, if less than 5 kPa, shunting due to pulmonary hypertension or CHD is likely. A raised $PaCO_2$ suggests a respiratory cause. This test is not diagnostic, but indicates which line of investigation should be pursued, e.g. echocardiography, Doppler blood flow studies. Beware of worsening PaO_2, by the administration of 100% oxygen, due to the closure of the ductus as here the circulation is dependent on it remaining open (Table 3.3).

2 Persistent pulmonary hypertension (persistent fetal circulation, PFC)

Definition The shunting of blood away from the lungs via the ductus arteriosus and foramen ovale due to persistently raised pulmonary vascular resistance.

Incidence 1 in 1500 live births.

Aetiology Usually precipitated by hypoxic delivery, meconium aspiration, hypoglycaemia and maternal diabetes, polycythaemia, or sepsis.

Pathophysiology Hypoxia → pulmonary artery constriction, mediated by leukotrienes, products of arachidonic acid metabolism. (Prostaglandins are also produced from arachidonic acid, of which E_1 and prostacyclin (PGI_2) can reverse the vasoconstrictive effect.)

Presentation Cyanosis, tachypnoea within 24 h of birth, sometimes with very rapid deterioration.

Diagnosis Systolic murmur due to tricuspid incompetence, normal ECG, chest X-ray slightly oligaemic. Echo confirms normal heart.

Treatment

1 Hyperventilate to reduce CO_2 and so peripheral pulmonary arterial resistance, with as high an oxygen concentration as necessary.
   NB: Pulmonary blood flow is reduced by high intrathoracic pressures, so avoid high end-expiratory pressures and an inspiratory to expiratory ratio of greater than 1:1. Pancuronium paralysis is essential.
2 Correct metabolic acidosis with i.v. bicarbonate or THAM.
3 If hypoxaemia persists:

   i Tolazoline, an α-adrenergic blocker, works best when >7.20 pH. Give i.v., 1–2 mg/kg bolus, then continuous infusion of 0.5–2 mg/kg/h, with dopamine and plasma expanders ready to counteract systemic hypotension.
   ii PGI_2 via pulmonary artery catheter.
   iii Nitric oxide inhalation has become widely available, reducing the need for extracorporeal membrane oxygenation (ECMO).

Prognosis

Mortality 20–40%. Neurological abnormality in up to half of survivors.

3   Myocardial ischaemia

Due to hypoxia or hypoglycaemia causing shock. ECG: T wave inversion, ischaemic/infarct pattern. Chest X-ray: cardiomegaly, pulmonary oedema. Digitalize, diuretics, oxygen.

4   Arrhythmias

i   Supraventricular tachycardia

Atrial rate 240–300/minute.
Detected in utero or as attacks of dyspnoea, and/or pallor.

Cause 80% idiopathic; also in ASD, Ebstein's malformation, cardiomyopathy, mitral valve prolapse.

Pathophysiology Usually re-entry of electrical impulse via an aberrant pathway, leading to circular excitation (other less common causes: atrial flutter, ectopic atrial tachycardia). Wolff–Parkinson–White syndrome is the best known. ECG between attacks: short P-R <0.12 s; QRS >0.12 s and abnormal ventricular excitation shows as a slur, i.e. delta wave.

Treatment In utero give mother digoxin.
   After birth: ice bag to face is effective in 90% (vagal stimulation), then try i.v. adenosine (short acting, safe) or cardioversion.
   Prophylaxis: oral digoxin (50% success), or oral flecainide.
   Hazards:

   a. Avoid digoxin in WPW (i.e. delta wave on ECG) which may precipitate ventricular tachycardia.

b. Verapamil can cause dangerous/fatal hypotension in infancy, or any patient in heart failure.

Prognosis 75% free of recurrence if age <3 months at onset.

ii Ventricular tachycardia

Uncommon in children, usually the result of electrolyte imbalance or structural heart disease.

iii Complete heart block

Causes: Most are idiopathic congenital. Corrected TGA or maternal lupus erythematosus must be considered in the newborn.

Heart failure and syncope occur if the rate falls below 50/min. If still in utero, deliver early; after birth consider a pacemaker.

5 Other causes of cyanosis and respiratory distress

- Septic shock.
- Seizures, CNS depression by drugs, trauma, asphyxia.
- Reye's syndrome, inborn metabolic error.
- Hypoglycaemia.

Management principles

1 Neonate

Early diagnosis improves prognosis. Ductus arteriosus patency may be necessary for survival, until palliation or repair is achieved. To facilitate this, early referral to a specialist centre in optimal condition is the aim.

   i General: avoid hypoxia as this leads to acidosis, hypoglycaemia, and hypovolaemia. Maintain temperature. Hypothermia is common in cyanosis, acidosis and shock.

   ii Prostaglandin E (PGE) i.v./orally to keep ductus arteriosus open.

      Prostaglandin may induce apnoea (requiring IPPV), raise body temperature, cause seizure, or thrombocytopenia.

Table 3.3 Benefits of establishing/maintaining ductal patency in CHD

Lesion benefiting	*Pathophysiological mechanism*
Obstructive right heart: pulmonary or tricuspid atresia/stenosis	Pulmonary blood flow maintained until systemic-pulmonary shunt fashioned
Obstructive left heart: preductal coarctation, interrupted aortic arch, severe aortic stenosis, hypoplastic left heart	Renal perfusion is critical, otherwise profound irreversible metabolic acidosis develops
Transposition of the great vessels without a septal defect	Otherwise inadequate mixing of the systemic and pulmonary circulations

Dose: PGE_1 i.v. 0.003–0.005 μg/kg/min or orally PGE_2 25–50 μg/kg hourly, reducing to 2 hourly after a week's treatment.

Supplemental oxygen without PGE can close the ductus arteriosus and worsen hypoxia.

iii Bicarbonate, glucose, calcium as biochemically indicated.

iv Albumin, dobutamine/dopamine to counteract shock and improve cardiac output.

2   Infants and children

i General: prop up, 30% oxygen, nasogastric feeds in infants. Cool if a large shunt causes a rise in the metabolic rate.

ii Correct biochemical abnormalities: acidosis, hypoglycaemia, hypocalcaemia.

iii Medication:

  a. Antibiotic for respiratory infection.

  b. Sedation with phenobarbitone if restless. Opiates are avoided as being likely to depress respiration more, especially if already cyanosed.

  c. Hypovolaemic shock: colloid and electrolytes (see Hypotension).

  d. Congestive failure:

   Diuretics to reduce preload. Potassium supplements are also required if digoxin is administered; alternatively add spironolactone.

   Vasodilator: captopril by reducing the after-load is increasingly preferred to inotropic digoxin for a failing heart, especially if due to a high output state, e.g. VSD.

   Inotropes: dobutamine +/– dopamine in the acute situation, digoxin for sustained inotropic action.

   Digoxin fails to benefit lesions with outflow obstruction, e.g. aortic stenosis, Fallot's tetralogy, and should not be used.

Drug dosages

Captopril: 1 mg/kg 8 hourly, increasing to a maximum of 3 mg/kg/dose.

Digoxin: Digitalization dose: premature 15 μg/kg over 24 h, in older age groups 40 μg/kg over 24 h; 1/2 dose stat, 1/4 at 8 and 16 h. Maintenance 5–15 μg/kg daily. Therapeutic level 1–3 ng/ml.

Diuretics: frusemide 1–3 mg/kg/day, (potassium chloride 2 mmol/kg/day as supplement unless spironolactone (potassium sparing effect) is used). Hydrochlorthiazide 1–4 mg/kg/day, spironolactone 3 mg/kg/day. Dobutamine/dopamine 5–10 μg/kg/min.

3   Consider surgical options early

Surgical treatment indications

Required by 60% with CHD, 40% of these in the first year of life.

1 Palliative procedures are less favoured than before, as one-stage corrective procedures, e.g. arterial switch in TGA, can now be done from the neonatal period onwards.

   i Shunts to improve blood supply to the lungs, e.g. pulmonary atresia.
   ii Banding to reduce pulmonary blood supply, e.g. multiple muscular VSD.
   iii Balloon septostomies to improve mixing at atrial level in TGA if the arterial switch is not done (see TGA).

2 Corrective procedures:

   i Cardiopulmonary bypass. The operative risk is related to the condition, not the procedure.
   ii Balloon dilatation: treatment of choice in pulmonary valve stenosis, aortic valve stenosis, recoarctation of the aorta.
   iii Occlusive devices will increasingly be used, for their low morbidity and avoidance of surgery: double umbrella occluder in PDA >10 kg, clam occluder for ASD, and possibly for VSDs.
   iv Human cadaveric homograft valves for aortic and pulmonary valve replacement are preferred as they do not require anticoagulation and, unlike tissue valved conduits, are not prone to calcific deterioration. Aortic valve homografts may need replacing as children grow.

3 Transplantation: now 50% survival to 3 years.

   i Cardiac for cardiomyopathies, endocardial fibroelastosis, hypoplastic left heart syndrome.
   ii Cardiopulmonary for Eisenmenger syndrome and pulmonary hypertension, and for cystic fibrosis.

Long-term problems for survivors of operated CHD

1 Bacterial endocarditis.
2 Arrhythmias.
3 Progressive pulmonary vascular disease.
4 Myocardial failure.
5 Replacement of valves and conduits.
6 Advice on employment, genetic risk to offspring, pregnancy.

Further reading

Somerville J (1989) Congenital heart disease in the adolescent. *Archives of Disease in Childhood*, **64**, 771–773

COMMONER AND SELECTED CONGENITAL HEART CONDITIONS

Classify clinically as either *acyanotic* or *cyanotic* and whether *obstructive* or with *increased flow or shunt*.

1   Acyanotic obstructive

Pulmonary stenosis 8%, coarctation of the aorta and aortic stenosis 6% each, and hypoplastic left heart syndrome, which often incorporates the latter two conditions.

Pulmonary stenosis

Definition

Thickened, dome shaped valve with central hole.

Pathophysiology

Right ventricle may hypertrophy and the cavity thus become smaller, further reducing flow to the lungs.

The pressure gradient in mild stenosis commonly does not progress as the child grows, but worsens in severe stenosis.

Clinical

Initially asymptomatic even if the stenosis is severe. Dyspnoea and fatigue appear as severity and decompensation increase.

Cheeks have almost crimson patches, with peripheral cyanosis.

Centrally pink unless a right to left shunt develops through a stretched (from back pressure in the right atrium) foramen ovale.

Low cardiac output is a sign of decompensation, so look for giant 'a' waves in the neck, liver enlargement and presystolic pulsation.

Palpation: right ventricular heave, systolic thrill second interspace, proportional to stenosis.

Heart sounds: the first is followed by a click as the valve opens, and the earlier it is, the tighter the stenosis. The second sound pulmonary component is delayed and may disappear if the stenosis is very severe.

Murmur: harsh loud ejection systolic, maximum second left interspace. The length increases proportional to the stenosis, i.e.:

Mild – ending before the second sound.

Severe – obliterating the second sound due to prolonged right ventricular systole.

Investigations

Chest X-ray: normal size heart, dilated pulmonary artery, diminished blood flow to the lungs.

ECG: right ventricular hypertrophy and peaked P waves develop.

Echo and Doppler show the anatomy and gradient, respectively.

Management

Doppler gradient <30 mmHg – no action; 30–50 mmHg – review; >50 mmHg – proceed to cardiac catheterization and consider balloon valvuloplasty. Right ventricular hypertrophy then subsides.

Coarctation of the aorta

Definition

Narrowing at the isthmus of the aorta due to ductal tissue in its wall. VSD and left heart valve abnormalities are common, and linked with other malformations, e.g. Turner's, congenital rubella.

1 Preducta.l Can be detected antenatally as a narrow aortic segment. Supply to the kidneys, liver and lower limbs is through the ductus until it closes. Thereafter circulation is maintained through a very narrow segment. Heart and renal failure, acidosis and hypoglycaemia follow, usually presenting in the first two weeks of life as the ductus closes.

Clinical signs Pallor, shock, poor femoral pulses and blood pressure. Always check using the right radial or brachial artery, as the left subclavian may be post coarctation.

BP normal in arms, low in legs.

Investigations X-ray chest: plethoric lung fields, dilated heart. ECG variable, left ventricular hypertrophy in severe stenosis.

Echo: shows the coarctation. Always look for VSD, and valvular abnormalities. Catheterization is now rarely indicated.

Management

i Medical emergency. Prompt treatment saves lives. Prostaglandin E_2 infusion opens the ductus; also give alkali, glucose, calcium i.v. Combat heart and kidney failure with diuretics and dopamine.

ii Surgical. Mortality improved by better medical management. The subclavian artery is incorporated into a flap to enlarge the aorta. VSD managed according to size, may need pulmonary artery banding at the same time.

2 Postductal constriction is associated with the development of collaterals across the coarcted segment antenatally. Bicuspid aortic valve may be present.

Clinical signs Presents as weak femoral pulses in infancy or delayed pulsed in later childhood once collaterals are well developed. They may be felt and heard round the scapulae.

BP elevated in the arms. Left ventricular hypertrophy.

Investigations X-ray chest: Penetrated view shows 'figure 3' = aortic bulge, constriction and post-stenotic bulge; reversed on barium swallow. Rib notching from collaterals after 6 years old.

ECG: Left ventricular hypertrophy.

Echo: Establishes site of coarctation, and the presence of other lesions. Doppler demonstrates the pressure gradient.

Management Surgery: Mortality <1%. Hypertension may be reactive and settles quickly, or may be more persistent (consider re-coarctation and the need for balloon dilatation) and requires regular follow up for both types of coarctation.

Further reading

Leader (1991) Coarctation repair – the First Forty Years. *Lancet*, ii, 546

Aortic stenosis

Site: valvular, supravalvular (William's syndrome), and subvalvular (diaphragm, hypertrophic obstructive cardiomyopathy) (Figure 3.2).

Aortic valve stenosis

Isolated type Boys>girls. Commoner in Turner's syndrome and coarctation.

Pathology Mild to moderate severity: bicuspid valve is commonest. Severe: unicusp or non-cuspid, like a diaphragm with a hole.
Clinical presentation Infancy: heart failure, sudden death.
   Childhood: asymptomatic murmur or with dyspnoea, central chest pain, and exercise induced faints.
   Pulse: normal unless severe when it is small volume, 'plateau' type.
   Precordium: pulsation seen, systolic thrill felt at suprasternal notch.
   Heart sounds: click before first sound, due to mobile aortic valves. Followed by an ejection systolic murmur in the aortic area and up into the neck. The second sound may be normal if mild or moderately stenosed, but single or even reversed with increased splitting on expiration if severe.

Investigations Chest X-ray: post-stenotic dilatation.
   ECG: often unhelpful. May show left ventricular hypertrophy.
   Echo:

- Cross-sectional: valve cusps may be reduced in number, thickened, and show reduced movement.
- M mode: shows closure of bicuspid valve is eccentric, and size of left ventricle increased.
- Doppler demonstrates gradient. Mild = 20 mmHg, moderate = 50 mmHg, severe = 60–100 mmHg. Catheter studies are now rarely done.

Management

1   Restriction of physical activities in moderate stenosis avoids gross hypertrophy and the dangers of arrhythmias and sudden death. Follow-up is essential to assess the degree of left ventricular hypertrophy.
2   Balloon dilatation is the procedure of choice.
3   Surgical indications for aortic valvotomy.

   i   Failure of balloon dilatation of the stenosis.
   ii Neonatal presentation, i.e. severe.
   iii Heart failure or ischaemia detected in moderately severe stenosis.

Valve replacement is rare in childhood, considered for severe aortic regurgitation which may occur after balloon or surgical valvotomy. Complications of prosthetic valves are incompetence and failure to grow with the child.

Further reading

Salley R K (1991) Left ventricular outflow tract obstruction in children. *Cardiology Clinics*, **9**, 381–396

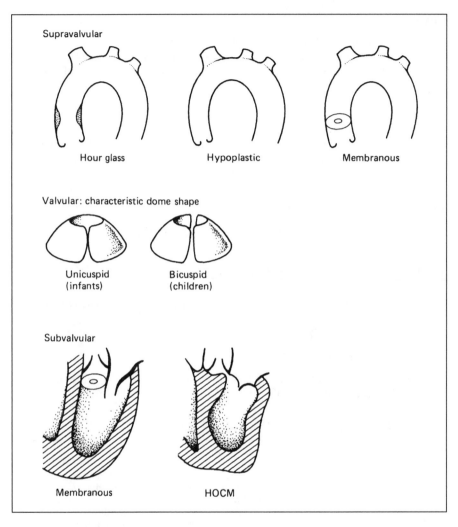

Figure 3.2 Aortic stenosis. Supravalvular: hourglass, hypoplastic, membranous. Valvular: unicuspid (infants), bicuspid (children). Subvalvular: membranous, hypertrophic obstructive cardiomyopathy (HOCM)

Hypoplastic left heart syndrome

Definition

Underdevelopment that affects the aorta mainly, but also left ventricle and its valves.

Incidence

Accounts for 25% of first week deaths from CHD.

Clinical

Life is sustained by the patency of the ductus arteriosus. Symptoms of dyspnoea, shock, and cyanosis develop at 1–5 days as it closes.

Differential diagnosis includes septicaemia and inborn errors of metabolism.

Management

Surgery, other than transplantation, has little to offer. Palliation, in which the Norwood procedure couples the right ventricle to the aorta, followed by the Fontan procedure in childhood, is generally not favoured in the UK.

Prognosis

Death within one week, rarely delayed to 2–3 months.

2 Acyanotic shunt from left to right

Ventriculoseptal defect 30%; persistent patent ductus arteriosus (PDA) 8%; atrioseptal defect (ASD) 8%.

Ventricular septal defect (VSD)

The commonest congenital cardiac abnormality (Figure 3.3; Table 3.4); 20% have an associated major malformation/chromosomal abnormality.

Table 3.4 Types of ventricular septal defect (VSD)

Type of defect	Natural history
1 *Muscular*: single hole or, if trabeculated, may be multiple	i Large defects: 75% close spontaneously or become smaller. Only 25% need surgery ii Small defects: All close, most by 2 years. Only risk is bacterial endocarditis
2 *Perimembranous* involving interventricular membrane +/– muscular defect	Spontaneous closure is less common than for muscular VSD as it is mainly a connective tissue defect extending into muscle i All are close to the tricuspid valve: the defect is made functionally smaller in 50% by valve tissue sticking to VSD margins = 'pseudoaneurysms' ii Remainder: if many small VSDs they are left, as long as there is no risk of pulmonary vascular disease
3 *Doubly committed subarterial* Muscular defects just below both valves	The VSD is usually large; always needs surgery as the aortic valve prolapses into the defect

Indications for VSD surgery

Dependent on (i) position and size of defect (ii) likelihood of spontaneous closure (iii) pulmonary blood flow and pulmonary vascular resistance.

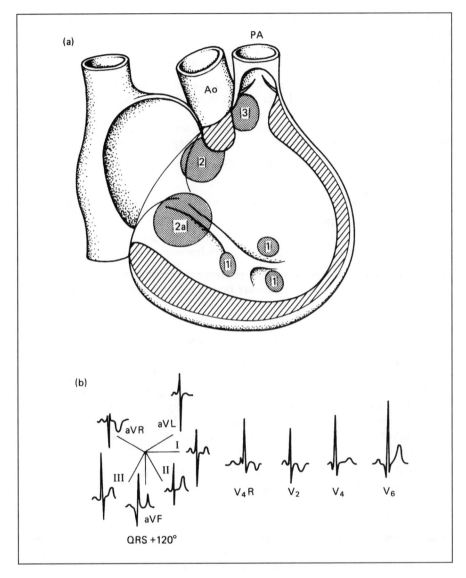

Figure 3.3
(a) Ventricular septal defect, viewed from the right side of the heart. 1 = muscular defect; 2 = perimembranous; 2a = large perimembranous; 3 = doubly committed subarterial. (b) ECG in VSD. Biventricular hypertrophy, R + S wave >70 mm, with right bundle branch block

Clinical situations

1 Asymptomatic small VSD. Most are muscular, so spontaneous closure is likely. Thrill is usually absent, pansystolic murmur best heard at apex, through to the lower back.

2   Moderate to large VSD. Dyspnoea, failure to thrive, recurrent chest infection, heart failure from 2–12 weeks old, as pulmonary vascular resistance falls. Thrill in the third left interspace, harsh pansystolic murmur. Presence of a mid-diastolic murmur indicates a 2:1 pulmonary:systemic shunt.

Investigations   Chest X-ray shows enlarged heart and pulmonary artery, increased vascularity both of hila and at periphery of lung fields.
ECG: biventricular hypertrophy.
Echo shows defect, and pseudoaneurysms are well seen. Doppler shows high flow L → R, low pressure gradient between ventricles.

Management   Persistent high blood flow may cause pulmonary vascular disease, so:

   i   Indications for corrective surgery in a symptomatic infant are:

     a. Failure to thrive.
     b. Persistently raised pulmonary artery pressure.
     c. Calculated shunt ratio of >2:1 pulmonary:systemic circulation.

   ii Pulmonary artery banding is preferred for multiple muscular VSDs, as early corrective surgery may be riskier, and they may close spontaneously anyway.

3   Large VSD with raised pulmonary vascular resistance.

   i   Common in Down's syndrome, and late presentation of large VSDs.
   ii   Early symptoms of heart failure resolve, so child seems well.
   iii Normal left ventricle, and a hard working right ventricle in which the pressure rises towards systemic, thus no thrill; presence of an ejection systolic murmur, and a loud single second heart sound.
   iv   Reversal of the shunt occurs eventually = cyanosis = *Eisenmenger syndrome of irreversible pulmonary hypertension.*

Investigations   Chest X-ray: Pulmonary vessel 'pruning' = reduced vascularity at the periphery of the lungs.
ECG: Right ventricular hypertrophy.
Echo: Large defect. Left to right shunt.

Management   Surgery is contraindicated if the pulmonary vascular resistance is elevated to >8 units, as measured at cardiac catheterization. Heart-lung transplant is the long-term alternative in selected cases.

Further reading

Trowitzsch E, Braun W, Stute M, Pielmeier W (1990) Diagnosis, therapy, and outcome of ventricular septal defects in the 1st year of life: a two-dimensional colour-Doppler echocardiography study. *European Journal of Pediatrics*, **149**, 758–761

Patent ductus arteriosus (PDA)

Normal functional closure occurs within hours of birth. May reopen with hypoxia and excess fluid administration (Table 3.5).

Auscultation

Like the symptoms, dependent on ductal size:

1 Small to medium.
   Thrill in the second left interspace, the classic continuous murmur due to a pressure gradient between the aorta and pulmonary artery throughout the cardiac cycle. The murmur persists on lying down, whereas a venous hum disappears.
      The second sound is loud, with both components close together.
2 Large, with raised pulmonary artery pressure due to high flow. Absent thrill, murmur present in systole only, and the characteristic one found in the preterm and term infant. The pressures in the aorta and pulmonary artery in diastole are equal, so no flow can occur then, but a mid-diastolic flow murmur through the mitral valve (increased return to left atrium) may be heard. The second heart sound is loud and single.

Table 3.5 Features of patent ductus arteriosus

	Term infants and older	*Prematures*
Incidence	1 in 2000	Up to 40% in <1500 g
Spontaneous closure	Rare after 2 weeks old	Usually by 3 months old
Clinical		Age 3–7 days stiff wet lungs with:
1 Small: asymptomatic. Normal pulses, BP		i Respiratory distress syndrome,
2 Medium: Tires easily, short stature. Pulse pressure wide, cardiomegaly		unable to wean off ventilator, or
3 Large: Failure to thrive, dyspnoea with feeds		ii Rapid respirations. Both show
		iii Heart failure with liver enlarged
Complications		
Heart failure, Eisenmenger syndrome, bacterial endocarditis		Ventricular haemorrhage, bronchopulmonary dysplasia, intractable heart failure

Investigations

Chest X-ray: cardiomegaly and enlarged pulmonary vessels.
   ECG: Left>right ventricular hypertrophy.
   Echo: confirms patency and Doppler shows the direction of flow. In prematures if the left atrial diameter is 1.5 × larger than aorta = large ductus.

Management

Term. Surgical ligation, or umbrella occluder at cardiac catheterization. Leave if pulmonary vascular disease is established, i.e. intervention is too late.

Preterm. Medical if <10 days old, <34 weeks' gestation. Indomethacin, fluid restriction + diuretic for heart failure. Delay if sepsis, bleeding, hyperbilirubinaemia, or renal dysfunction. Closure effective in up to 80%.
   Surgery if no response or older.

Prognosis

Term.   Large PDA without surgery 50% dead by middle age.
Operation <1% mortality.
Small PDA: main risk is endocarditis.
Preterm.   Without treatment 30% die.

Atrioseptal defect (ASD)

Definitions

Defects of the septum may be:

1   Simple, involving the interatrial septum alone = ostium secundum
2   Complex = atrioventricular septal defect (AVSD) which is either:

   i   Partial (ostium primum) if no ventricular component. The mitral valve is usually cleft.
   ii Complete if a large central defect due to an ASD and VSD with a single large atrioventricular valve. Cyanosis usually supervenes because of pulmonary vascular disease. Down's syndrome accounts for 50%, and occurs in 80% of Down's with CHD.

Pathophysiology

1   Flow is L → R, secondary to the fall in pulmonary vascular resistance, into the low resistance right heart. Further contributions to flow often occur:

   i   One or more anomalous pulmonary veins are often present, draining into the right atrium (sinus venosus defect).
   ii Primum/AVSD defects: may result in mitral regurgitation producing a pansystolic apical murmur. Complete defects are prone to irreversible pulmonary hypertension in childhood.

2   Murmurs are due to increased flow across the valves, not the ASD itself.

   i   Across pulmonary valve → ejection systolic.
   ii Across tricuspid valve → mid-diastolic if >2:1 shunt. The murmur increases on inspiration.

3   Fixed splitting of the second heart sound: the increased volume causes prolonged contraction time of the right ventricle.

Clinical

Ostium secundum

1   Symptoms rare in childhood. Only in a very large ASD, then like a primum defect.
    Adults: heart failure, pulmonary hypertension, atrial fibrillation.
2   May be tall, long fingers and toes.
3   Right ventricular heave.

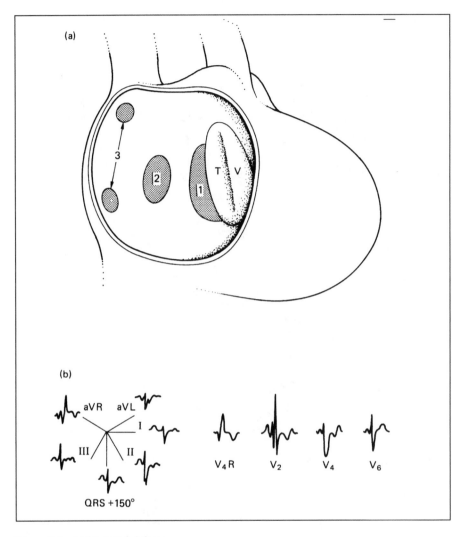

Figure 3.4 Atrial septal defects
(a) Anatomy: view of the right atrium
    1 = ostium primum
    2 = ostium secundum
    3 = sinus venosus defect
    TV = tricuspid valve
(b) ECG in ostium secundum defect, with peaked P waves in leads II, V_2, right bundle branch block, and right ventricular hypertrophy
(c) ECG in ostium primum showing biventricular hypertrophy, (unusual unless pulmonary vascular disease is present) right bundle branch block and prolonged P-R interval. (Often shows a superior axis)
(d) Complete atrioventricular septal defect. View from the left side of the heart
    1 = ASD in the lowest part of the atrial septum
    2 = common atrioventricular valve in closed position
    3 = subvalvular VSD
(e) Surgical repair, of a complete AVSD, with corresponding patches, and reconstruction of the valve into two or replaced by homografts

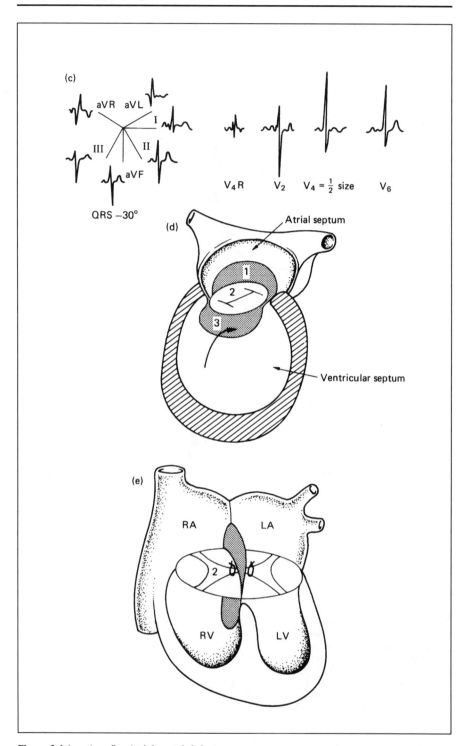

Figure 3.4 (*continued*)   Atrial septal defects

Atrioventricular septal defect

1 Severity of mitral incompetence determines:

i Symptoms: 50% dyspnoea, tired, frequent chest infections.
ii Prognosis: Poor without surgery.

2 Often short, Harrison's sulci, bulging precordium.
3 Both ventricles enlarged in complete defects.
4 Heart sounds and murmurs similar for both, plus mitral incompetence murmur in secundum (not loud) type.

Although a murmur in the pulmonary area may suggest an ASD, a variable splitting of the second heart sound excludes it.

Investigations

Ostium secundum

ECG: Right axis 90–160°, partial right bundle branch block pattern (RBBB).
Chest X-ray: Prominent pulmonary arteries and vessels to periphery.
Doppler: Flow shows size of shunt.

Atrioventricular septal defect. Left axis –60 to –180°, similar RBBB but more right ventricular hypertrophy = rsR in V_4R, V_1 and tall/bifid P waves, PR prolonged.
Cardiomegaly more likely.
Shunt, and mitral regurgitation also present.

Surgery

Ostium secundum. Close if shunt >2:1, at 4 years old. Clam occluder is an alternative to surgery. Mortality <0.5%.

Atrioventricular septal defect. Partial atrioventricular septal defect (AVSD) closed before school age. Mortality 1%. Complete AVSD usually needs correction in infancy to avoid pulmonary vascular damage. Mortality 10–20%.

Further reading

Rome J J, Keane J F, Perry S B, Spevak P J, Lock J E (1990) Double-umbrella closure of atrial defects. Initial clinical applications. *Circulation*, **82**, 751–758.

3 Cyanotic obstructive, i.e. *reduced* pulmonary blood flow

Fallot's tetralogy 6%, single ventricle with tricuspid atresia 2%, Ebstein's malformation, pulmonary atresia <1%.

Fallot's tetralogy

Pulmonary stenosis, large VSD, overriding of the aorta and secondary right ventricular hypertrophy (Figure 3.5).

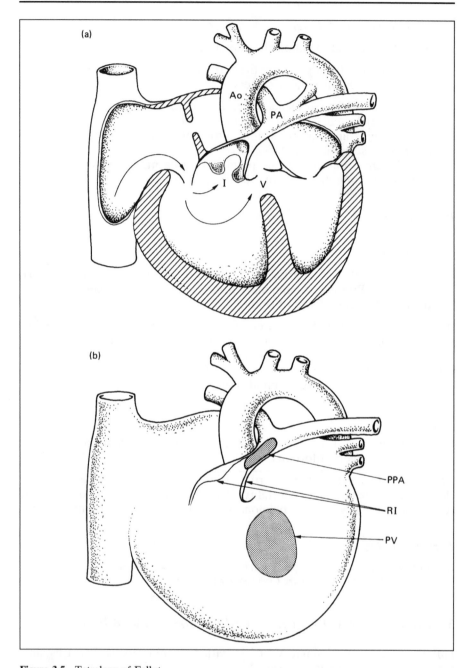

Figure 3.5   Tetralogy of Fallot
(a) Anatomy. I = infundibular narrowing plus pulmonary stenosis. Ao = aorta, PA =
      pulmonary artery, V = VSD
(b) Surgical correction. PPA = patched pulmonary artery +/- homograft valve
      RI = resected infundibular muscle
      PV = patched VSD
(c) ECG shows right ventricular hypertrophy and marked right axis deviation

Figure 3.5 (*continued*)   Tetralogy of Fallot

Pathophysiology

The degree of infundibular pulmonary stenosis determines the severity. The right ventricular hypertrophy is secondary to the systemic pressure from continuity with the overriding aorta.

Cyanosis appears:

  i From birth if effectively pulmonary atresia, depending on ductus arteriosus and its closure.
 ii From 4–6 months old, 'cyanotic spells' due to infundibular spasm as this portion becomes more narrow as the child grows.
iii After exercise → squatting: reduces blood flow to and from the lower limbs, raises systemic BP and oxygen saturation.

Findings include:

  i Poor growth proportional to cyanosis.
 ii Clubbing.
iii Cardiac: right ventricular heave, single second heart sound. Murmurs of ventricular defect and pulmonary stenosis may disappear during cyanotic spells due to infundibular spasm, when the pulmonary outlet is obstructed. Heart failure is rare.

Complications

1 Hypoxic attacks can result in brain damage and death.
2 Cerebral thromboses due to high haematocrit, risk increased by dehydration or iron deficiency anaemia (hypochromic RBCs are less deformable).
3 Bacterial endocarditis.
4 Cerebral abscess may be secondary to 2, not 3.

Investigations

See ECG. Chest X-ray: 'boot-shaped' heart in only 50%, right-sided aorta 20%. Echo confirms. Cardiac catheterization only if pulmonary artery branch stenoses are suspected.

Management

1   Hypoxic episodes require:

   i   Knee-elbow position.
   ii Oxygen.
   iii Drugs – morphine + propranolol to ease infundibular spasm, bicar-bonate for acidosis. Noradrenaline if unresponsive to propranolol (raises systemic resistance). Digoxin is contraindicated. Early opera-tion is mandated.

2   Surgery.

   i   Early systemic to pulmonary shunt (e.g. Blalock) may be required for severe pulmonary stenosis.
   ii Correction of the outflow tract obstruction, sometimes with a patch through the outflow tract and valve (transannular patch).
   iii Patch the VSD.

Prognosis

Presurgery 30% dead by one year, 75% by 10 years. With surgery 90% survive to adult life, and 90% of them have a normal lifestyle.

Single ventricle with tricuspid atresia

Blood flows from the right atrium through the patent foramen ovale to the left heart, and then through a VSD to the pulmonary artery (Figure 3.6a).
   ECG: uncharacteristic left heart predominance in the newborn period.
   Surgery: palliative shunt initially, followed by the Fontan procedure where feasible (Figure 3.6b).

Ebstein's anomaly

Definition

'Atrialization' of the right ventricle by posterior and septal leaflets of the tricuspid valve attached to the endocardium below the valve's fibrous ring.

Clinical and investigations

Obstruction to flow to the lungs and dilatation of the right atrium result, seen on chest X-ray and echo. The ECG is characteristic, with tall P waves, right bundle branch pattern. Paroxysmal tachycardia or atrial flutter are typical arrhythmias.

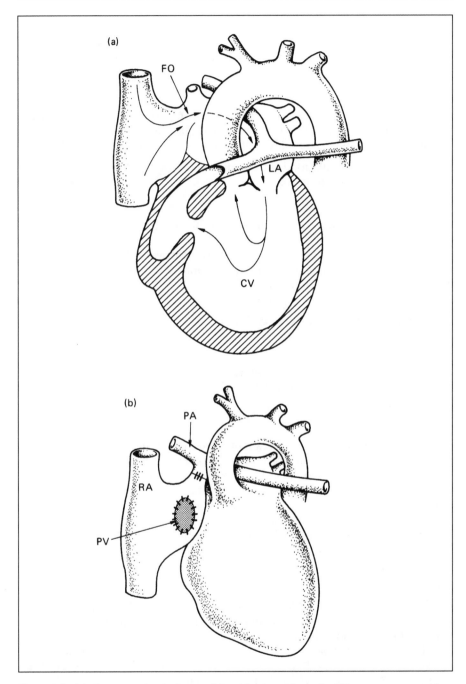

Figure 3.6   (a) Anatomy of a single ventricle with tricuspid atresia. CV = common ventricle,
LA = left atrium, FO = foramen ovale
(b) Surgical correction, the Fontan procedure connecting the right atrium to pulmonary
artery, disconnecting it from the right ventricle. PA = pulmonary artery, RA = right atrium,
PV = patched VSD

Management

Conservative: if pulmonary stenosis is associated consider a shunt. Surgical reconstruction of the tricuspid valve carries a high risk.

Pulmonary atresia

1   With intact interventricular septum – incompatible with life unless the ductus remains patent. The Fontan procedure may be effective.
2   With VSD: similar to Fallot's tetralogy, cyanosis presenting earlier.

The pulmonary circulation is often abnormal, supplied by collaterals which are surgically difficult to correct.

4   Cyanotic with *increased* pulmonary blood flow

Transposition of great vessels, complete atrioventricular (AV) defect (previously called AV canal or endocardial cushion defect) 4% each, and total anomalous pulmonary venous connection.

Transposition of the great vessels (TGA)

Definition

The aorta is attached to the anatomic right ventricle, the pulmonary artery to the anatomic left ventricle (Figure 3.7).

Pathophysiology

Circulations are in parallel instead of in series. If the only connection is through the ductus arteriosus and/or a patent foramen ovale, cyanosis inevitably follows as it closes, unless a VSD is present.

Clinical

Cyanosis within 24 h of birth. No dyspnoea, and a murmur is often absent. Progressive metabolic acidosis.

Investigations

Chest X-ray: 'egg on side' due to a narrow vascular pedicle. May be obscured by the thymus initially, which involutes rapidly due to cyanosis or stress.
    ECG: Often normal, later right ventricular hypertrophy.
    Echo: Abnormal anatomical relationship of the two great vessels which are in parallel instead of winding round each other. The aorta lies in front of the pulmonary artery, i.e. a reversal of the normal.

Management

1   Prostaglandin infusion, support pH with alkali.

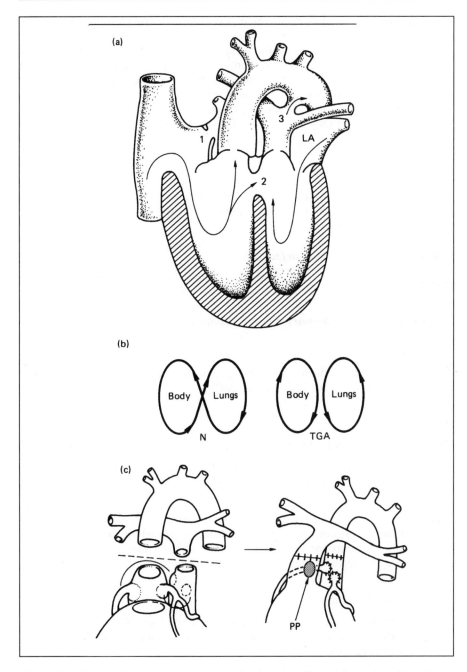

Figure 3.7 Transposition of the great arteries. (a) Anatomy. Potential sites for mixing 1 = foramen ovale, 2 = VSD, 3 = PDA
(b) Circulation
   N = normal; TGA = transposition
(c) Surgical arterial 'switch'
   PP = pericardial patch to where coronary arteries have been removed

Avoid additional oxygen which may hasten ductal closure, with consequent worsening of hypoxia.

2   Direct arterial 'switch' as the first procedure, of the aorta, with the coronary arteries, to the left ventricle, pulmonary artery to the right ventricle. This correction allows the right ventricle to pump at low pressures and is considered more physiological than the previously preferred balloon septostomy followed by the atrial baffle operation of Mustard or Senning at 6–9 months old. Switch is also the preferred operation if a VSD is present.

Prognosis

Before surgery was available mortality was 80% by 1 year, now 80% survival to adult life is predicted. Operative mortality in the best units is 5%.

Complete atrioventricular defect

See ASD.

Total anomalous pulmonary venous connection (TAPVC)

Definition

The pulmonary veins drain into the right heart not the left atrium. Flow is obstructed or non-obstructed (Figure 3.8).

Pathophysiology

Obligatory right to left shunt → pulmonary congestion with cyanosis:

  i   Proportional to the shunt through the stretched foramen ovale.
  ii Most severe in obstructed TAPVC, which is typically infradiaphragmatic.

In the newborn it may present as respiratory distress syndrome with no improvement despite oxygen administration, or persistent tachypnoea.

Obstruction due to narrowing of the veins at insertion is invariable in the infradiaphragmatic type, causing pulmonary hypertension.

Non-obstructed drainage

  i   Supracardiac via the innominate = 'cottage loaf' X-ray appearance.
  ii Cardiac via the sinus venosus or the coronary sinus. Both present later, in cardiac failure.

Investigation

Difficult to diagnose on echo. An inexperienced echocardiographer may miss the abnormal pulmonary vein connections and misdiagnose as a hypoplastic left heart, or normal if the left ventricle is a good size.

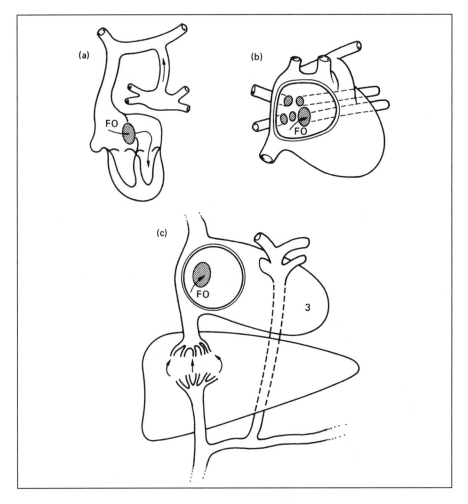

Figure 3.8 Total anomalous pulmonary venous connection. FO = foramen ovale
(a) Supracardiac via the left innominate vein
(b) Cardiac. The pulmonary veins drain into the right atrium
(c) Infradiaphragmatic via the portal vein

Surgery

Correction is usually urgent.

Mortality 80% without surgery. With surgery 5–30%, depending on age, severity of acidosis, type of obstruction and size of the left ventricle.

INFLAMMATORY HEART DISEASE

Cardiac failure due to bacterial and viral infection, or rheumatic heart disease.

Infective endocarditis

Definition

Bacterial infection occurring at sites of endothelial damage where a jet of blood impinges.

Uncommon in infants, the risk is increased in cyanotic conditions, and after cardiac surgery. *Streptococcus viridans* and *Staphylococcus aureus* are the main pathogens.

Clinical

Fever, pallor, arthralgia, splenomegaly, heart failure, and signs of emboli (haematuria, splinter haemorrhages, hemiplegia, pleurisy).

Prior treatment with antibiotic obscures classic signs, so a high index of suspicion is needed to avoid heart damage, or death (still 25%).

Management

Start treatment as soon as blood cultures have been taken (4 in the first 24 h, 2 in the next 24 h).

Penicillin + aminoglycoside for 6 weeks, adjusted according to microbial culture and sensitivities. High bactericidal levels are required.

Prophylaxis

Maintain good oral hygiene and dental care. Fluoride supplements are helpful.
   Antibiotic cover indicated for:

   i   All congenital heart lesions, and always continued for life after cardiac surgical repair (except for a ligated PDA, secundum ASD or spontaneous closure of a VSD).
   ii Acquired: rheumatic heart disease, previous infective endocarditis, acquired valve disease.
   iii Hypertrophic cardiomyopathy, arteriovenous fistulae.

Procedures and recommended antibiotics

1   Dental treatment and operations to the upper respiratory tract: *Streptococcus viridans* is common so give amoxycillin orally/i.m. one hour before treatment 3 g, or 1.5 g if <10 years old.
   For penicillin allergy, erythromycin 1 g orally, or 0.5 g if <10 years old, or clindamycin 6 mg/kg.
2   Surgery to gut and renal tract: enterococci common, so give gentamicin 2 mg/kg + ampicillin, 0.5 g under 10 years, 1 g thereafter, both i.m.
3   Prosthetic heart valves best protected by i.m. ampicillin + flucloxacillin, 0.5 g under 10 years, 1 g thereafter, of each, before treatment and at 8 and 16 h after.

Acute myocarditis

Definition

Acute heart failure after a prodromal illness. Usually viral, e.g. Coxsackie, ECHO, influenza, mumps.

Investigations

Echo: dilated heart, reduced ejection fraction.
  ECG: low voltage pattern, arrhythmias, injury as Q waves.

Differential diagnosis

Septicaemia, meningococcal septicaemia, rheumatic fever, Kawasaki disease, anomalous left coronary artery (arising from the pulmonary artery, causes angina and death).

Treatment

Digoxin, diuretics, oxygen.

Prognosis

Recovery 80%, some die, others go on to endocardial fibroelastosis. Neonatal coxsackie B myocarditis has an 80% mortality.

Hypertrophic obstructive cardiomyopathy (HOCM) AD

Definition

Excessive progressive thickening of the left ventricular wall leads to stiffness with poor diastolic filling, and obstruction to outflow.

Clinical

Dyspnoea, chest pain, syncope, sudden death from arrhythmias.

* Double peak to the pulse is pathognomonic, and due to interruption of systolic ejection by septal obstruction.
* Apex beat thrusting, with a double impulse. Mitral regurgitation murmur is heard in some.
  ECG: left ventricular hypertrophy, occasionally with Q waves.
  Echo: thickening of interventricular septum.

Management

Beta blockers or calcium channel antagonists prevent symptoms, and may possibly reverse hypertrophy. Important cause of sudden death in young athletes, so advise against sporting activities.

Endocardial fibroelastosis

Definition

Considered to be the end stage of viral myocarditis or dilated cardiomyopathy.

Pathophysiology

Thickened white endocardium lining a dilated underfunctioning left ventricle, as opposed to the contracted type seen with hypoplastic left heart or secondary obstruction to the left ventricle.

Clinical

Peak age 6 months. May have a regurgitant pansystolic murmur due to gross dilatation of the left heart.

Investigations

Echo: Dilated left ventricle, ejection fraction a third of normal.
   ECG: Left ventricular hypertrophy.
   Chest X-ray: Cardiomegaly.

Treatment and prognosis

As for acute myocarditis. Heart transplant for intractable cases.

Rheumatic fever (RF)

Definition

An autoimmune reaction after a group A β-haemolytic streptococcal pharyngitis, involving skin, joints, the heart and its valves, and the brain.

Incidence

Falling in developed countries to 0.01% compared with up to 1% in Third World urban poverty. Recent upsurge in cases in the USA.

Risk in the UK

1 in 30 000 group A β-haemolytic streptococcal infections, a fall from 1 in 300 in 1960; 16 children affected in 1990 (reported to the British Paediatric Surveillance Unit).

Pathophysiology

Cross reaction between a genetically susceptible person's antibodies to streptococcal wall antigen (Lancefield group A) and their own heart, synovial or brain tissues. Family history of RF is common.

Round cells, giant cells and plasma cells, often contained in Aschoff nodules, characterize the inflammatory reaction, except in the brain where the inflammation in chorea is non-specific.

Clinical

Onset: Rare <3 years old, 10–21 days after a streptococcal sore throat/infection. Abdominal pain may precede the following:

1   Arthritis with fever (75%). Large joints are swollen, hot, and painful on movement. Different joints become involved day to day, rarely more than three at a time. Duration 3–4 weeks, resolve completely.
    Mild arthralgia is a commoner presentation, when RF is less easy to diagnose.
2   Carditis. Affects 50%. As part of an arthritis or non-specific illness, with evening fever, weight loss, poor appetite, cough and dyspnoea.
    Pulse: tachycardia, raised sleeping pulse rate. Bradycardia occasionally.
    Cardiomegaly. Heart failure may occur. Pericardial friction rub is rare. Heart sounds become muffled, with tic-tac or gallop rhythm.
    Murmurs:
    Apical
    systolic, high pitched (mitral incompetence, chordae stretched).
    mid-diastolic Carey Coombes (mitral orifice narrowing due to swollen valve leaflets).
    Left sternal edge – early diastolic of aortic incompetence.
3   Rheumatic nodules in 1%, over pressure points. Non tender, containing Aschoff nodules, develop weeks later.
4   Skin rashes. Erythema marginatum, a serpigenous outline which varies over the day, and erythema nodosum, are both found in other conditions.
5   Sydenham's chorea (St Vitus' dance) 15%.
    Onset gradual, 5–15 years old. Girls>boys, carditis in 25%.

Investigations

1   Antistreptolysin O titre raised, streptococci on culture. ESR raised.
2   ECG: prolonged P-R (>0.2 s), Wenkebach phenomenon.
3   Echo: small pericardial effusion, dilatation and reduced contractility of the left ventricle, stretched chordae of the mitral valve.

Diagnosis

A useful aid to avoid overdiagnosis is Jones' criteria:

1   Major manifestations, a total of 5 (above).
2   Minor manifestations (raised ESR, fever, arthralgia, previous RF or rheumatic heart disease, prolonged P-R).
3   Supportive: recent scarlet fever, rising ASOT, streptococci on culture.
RF = 2 major or 1 major + 2 minor + preceding streptococcal infection.
Some cases of RF do not fulfil these criteria, especially if seen early.

Differential diagnosis

1   Arthritis. Conditions commonly confused are:

   i   Growing pains: acute pain in leg muscles causes nocturnal waking, often with tears. No fever, normal ESR, joints and heart.
   ii Still's disease: <5 years, fever is diurnal, with maculopapular rash; small joints are often involved, and hepatosplenomegaly and lymphadenopathy, not just liver; pericarditis alone, not pancarditis.
   iii Henoch-Schönlein purpura: any age over 1 year, often no fever, rash is urticarial → purpuric, affects large and small joints. Acute abdominal pain and haematuria are common.

2   Murmurs: characteristics of functional murmurs differ.
3   Chorea.

Management

Penicillin, erythromycin or cephalexin for 10 days.

Bed rest for painful joints, aspirin 120 mg/kg/day for 14 days, then halved until arthritis and fever have settled.

Presence of mitral incompetence or ventricular dilatation are an indication for restriction to bed or chair. Steroids are only indicated for heart failure or complete heart block, as rebound on stopping is usual. Limit to bed or chair until ESR <20 mm. Full sporting activities after 6 months.

Chorea – as for RF. Reduction of movements achieved with haloperidol.

Prevention of recurrence with daily penicillin or erythromycin 250 mg twice daily, probably for life. Follow up is essential to monitor for valvular damage and the taking of antibiotic.

Prognosis

Death from acute and chronic rheumatic heart disease is 2% in childhood.

Chronic rheumatic heart disease occurs in 30% after acute RF.

* Repeated attacks of RF are more likely in these children.
* Severity of valvular damage is related to the number of attacks of RF.
* Mitral and aortic valve damage: mitral stenosis is the commonest sequela.

Further reading

Gillette P C (ed) (1990) Congenital heart disease. *Pediatric Clinics of North America*, **37**, no.1
Jordan S C, Scott O (1989) *Heart Disease in Paediatrics*. 3rd edn. Butterworths: London
Long W A (1990) *Fetal and Neonatal Cardiology*. Saunders:Philadelphia (for excellent explanations of the physiology and cardiac surgery)
Kavey R W, Kaplan E L (1989) Resurgence of acute rheumatic fever. *Pediatrics*, **84**, 585–586

Index